No More MOO

The Dairy-Free
and Lactose-Free Guide
to Living Well with Lactose
Intolerance

Savannah Paris

REGENCY
Publications

No More MOO

ISBN-13: 978-1489582874

ISBN-10: 1489582878

Contents

Soups   140

Entrees & Sides   159

Desserts 231

Chapter 2: Causes of leay gut   311

Introduction
My Story

All I had to do was drive thirteen miles to get home—but I didn't make it.

The evening had begun innocently enough. As president of a professional writer's association, I was the host of our annual awards ceremony. As master of ceremonies, my job was to keep the audience entertained, move the show along and hand out awards to happy winners.

The event was held at an exclusive, upscale restaurant, which provided an appealing selection of appetizers and hors d'oeuvres. People hovered around the tables talking, eating, drinking and socializing.

Because I had to prepare for my hosting duties, I quickly choose two appetizers that looked appealing and took a few small bites. I worked for about a half hour behind the scenes. Just as I took my place on stage, I was stunned by a wave of stomach cramping that took my breath away.

The only thing I could think of was to get to a restroom, but then the spotlight was, literally, on me. Thankfully adrenaline kicked in and I began the show, which lasted for more than an hour. As soon as the show was over, my pumped-up adrenaline vanished and the painful cramping came back stronger than ever.

I found a restroom in time and, after an attack of diarrhea, the pain stopped. But unfortunately, as I started driving home, my stomach cramping returned in full force. Because I had just driven onto a long causeway (a raised highway bordered by water on both sides), there were no exits, no stops and no chance of finding a restroom.

The cramping got so bad I had difficulty pushing the gas pedal down. I felt nauseated and rapidly broke out in a cold sweat from the pain. My only goal was to get to a restroom as soon as possible. When I was finally able to exit the causeway, I spotted a restaurant and quickly pulled into the parking lot. This is extremely embarrassing to admit, but I didn't make it to the restroom in time.

That was my life with lactose intolerance. Apparently the small amount of hidden dairy in those few bites was enough to do me in that day.

I've written this book because I don't want this to be your life, too. I don't want you to suffer the discomfort and, sometimes, the humiliation of this distressing and often painful condition because *you don't have to*. Wherever you are on the lactose intolerance spectrum—from mild to severe, you can learn to live a symptom-free life and enjoy a lactose-free lifestyle.

Inside this book, you'll find the information and techniques I used to rid myself of the symptoms of lactose intolerance. Whether you suffer a little or a lot from lactose intolerance, **No More MOO** is written for you.

Why should I read this book?

To feel better.

If you suffer from lactose intolerance, or you just want to avoid dairy products for a healthier diet, this book is for you.

Millions of Americans suffer from lactose intolerance—some with severe, painful symptoms—but it doesn't have to be this way. Lactose intolerance can be controlled with a diary-free and lactose-free diet. You'll find a wealth of information in this book to help you make the important shift to living lactose free. With this knowledge, you can lead a healthier life and—most importantly—feel better.

Lactose-free living is a lifestyle, it's a diet, and it's a whole new way of looking at things—especially cooking.

What you'll learn:

PART ONE is full of information about lactose intolerance, lactose-free eating and the lactose-free lifestyle.

If you want basic information about lactose intolerance—its causes and its symptoms—read **Chapter One—Lactose 101**.

Chapter Two is all about correctly diagnosing lactose intolerance. You'll find that other diseases can mimic the symptoms of lactose intolerance, and why it's critical to get a correct diagnosis.

Wondering why you have lactose intolerance and others don't? You'll discover how prevalent lactose intolerance is, and some of the reasons why you may have become lactose intolerant in **Chapter Three—Why Me?**

In **Chapter Four**, you'll find out how to deal with mild to moderate lactose intolerance, including knowing what your personal lactose limit is, and discovering where to find hidden lactose. There's a section on eating out, and strategies to help you maintain an enjoyable lifestyle.

Chapter Five deals with severe lactose intolerance. You'll discover the sweeping lifestyle changes you need to make to feel better, and ways of coping and thriving with this new way of thinking about food. There's also an easy explanation of lactose intolerance to help you explain to loved ones why you can't eat dairy products, and strategies to get them to help you.

Chapter Six talks about the lactose-free kitchen, and offers methods to help you cook lactose-free.

Chapter Seven is all about the essential vitamins and minerals you need, and how to get them from food when you can't get them from milk and dairy.

Chapter Eight talks about supplements—how to find reputable ones, how much to take, and health frauds you should be aware of.

PART TWO offers an extensive cookbook with dozens of recipes ranging from lactose-free breakfasts to dinners, and lactose-free snacks to desserts. There are even recipes for shakes.

No More MOO is a comprehensive look at all aspects of lactose intolerance. Extensive research has gone into its writing to give you the best and most up-to-date information possible.

Chapter One
Lactose Intolerance 101

Got milk?

There's no shortage of milk in the United States and there's no shortage of people who love it. For many of us, it's unthinkable to have our coffee or morning cereal without milk. Yes, we love our milk—although, unfortunately, sometimes it doesn't love us.

If you suffer from mild to moderate lactose intolerance, milk and dairy products can produce unpleasant symptoms. If you suffer from severe lactose intolerance, like I did, milk and dairy are more than a little bothersome—they're the enemy—and they take no prisoners.

Lactose Defined

What is lactose anyway? Some people incorrectly believe that lactose is a form of fat that's found in dairy products and milk. Lactose is actually a sugar—not a fat. It's often referred to as a "natural sugar" because it's found specifically in milk that's produced by mammals.

If you eat dairy products, you're consuming lactose.

And you may not know this, but if you're eating and drinking alternative milk and dairy products, you're also consuming lactose. Any milk produced by a mammal will cause symptoms; so substituting other types of milk—such as goat's milk or sheep's milk—unfortunately, isn't the solution. Yogurt made from sheep's milk, for example, actually contains more lactose than cow's milk.

Important: lactose intolerance is **NOT** a milk allergy

Lactose intolerance is your intestine's reaction to milk **sugar**. A milk allergy is a systemic immune reaction against milk **proteins**.

Some symptoms of milk allergy can be similar to lactose intolerance symptoms. If you have any gastric symptoms, you could be lactose intolerant, have a milk allergy, or both.

You'll discover how to determine if you have a milk allergy and other important tests for determining lactose intolerance in Chapter Two.

The basics

First, here's some basic information:

Lactose intolerance—also known as "lactose malabsorption" or "lactase deficiency"—is a condition where the body is unable to digest lactose (milk sugar).

Lactose has two main components: *glucose* (the type of sugar your body can easily digest) and *galactose*. When you consume dairy products, your body is faced with the job of splitting lactose into these two components.

Got lactase?

Lactase, which is manufactured in the lining of the small intestine, is the only enzyme in your digestive system that can break down **lactose**.

Ideally, you should have enough **lactase** to continually and regularly break down and absorb **lactose**. But, if you're suffering from lactose intolerance this, regrettably, isn't the case.

What causes it?

There are three main types of lactose intolerance:

Primary lactose intolerance:

This is the most common form of the condition. The lactase gene expression turns off in childhood and, over time, your body can stop producing adequate amounts of this essential enzyme. It may take years for symptoms to appear, usually in adulthood.

Secondary lactose intolerance:

If you become ill from a disease that affects your small intestine—like inflammatory conditions, bacterial, viral, or parasitic infections—you can become lactose intolerant. Fortunately, in most cases, this lactose intolerance disappears in a few weeks.

Congenital lactase deficiency:

This is a rare case in which a baby is born without the ability to produce lactase. Infants born with this condition will remain lactose intolerant throughout their lives.

Note: Some *premature* infants are born lactose intolerant. But, this type of lactose intolerance is generally temporary. Once the baby's GI tract is more mature, he or she will begin producing a normal amount of lactase. At that point, the baby will be able to drink milk and other lactose products with no problems.

What happens when you don't have enough lactase?

How much dairy you can eat depends on how much lactase enzyme your body makes. If you have little or no lactase, your body labors when you eat lactose. The less lactase your body produces, the more severe your symptoms will be. If lactase isn't available in any form, your body will not be able to digest and absorb lactose.

So what happens when your body can't digest lactose? In short, when your body doesn't have enough lactase to thoroughly break down lactose in your small intestine, it reaches the large intestine intact. When this undigested material enters the large intestine, it serves as food for bacteria dwelling there. As the bacteria feed upon the undigested milk, sugar, gases and irritating acids are produced creating unpleasant and sometime severe symptoms.

What are the symptoms?

They're pretty much hard to ignore:

- Bloating

- Intestinal cramping

- Acute abdominal pain

- A stomach that gurgles

- Gas

- Diarrhea

- Vomiting

How do I know if what I have is lactose intolerance?

This is important. There may be other reasons why you could be experiencing some or all of these symptoms. There can be a number of *other* conditions you may be suffering from that aren't remotely related to lactose intolerance. That's why it's essential to know their cause. Don't guess; you need to be one hundred percent sure of what's actually affecting your health, and how to deal with it.

Chapter Two
Diagnosing Lactose Intolerance

You may be able to diagnose lactose intolerance yourself. The simplest test is called the "milk challenge" test.

The milk challenge testing process

The milk challenge is an easy way of diagnosing lactose intolerance. To take the test, you fast overnight, and then drink a glass of milk in the morning. After that, you have nothing to eat or drink for three to five hours. If you're lactose intolerant, the milk should produce symptoms within several hours of ingestion.

But this test may not be conclusive. If you're not sure, you can choose to try the next test—dairy elimination.

Dairy elimination test

Try eliminating all sources of dairy products and other products that may contain lactose for one to two weeks. Believe me; I understand this is no ordinary undertaking.

To test myself, I eliminated all dairy and processed foods, ate only vegetables and meat, and drank soy milk for two weeks. (I knew for sure these items didn't contain lactose.) My symptoms went away.

To reintroduce dairy, I ate a big bowl of my favorite chocolate ice cream. I didn't know it at the time, but many ice cream manufacturers add additional lactose to ice cream to make it creamier. Wow, it didn't take long. My lactose intolerance symptoms came back in less than an hour. I decided I didn't need to pursue any further testing. Without a doubt, I was sure I was lactose intolerant.

If this one- to two-week regimen of just meat, vegetables and a milk alternative (such as soy or almond milk) is too difficult for you, you can try a less restricted diet. But, if you decide to go for this self-test, it will take some detective work on your part to eliminate all dairy products. Dairy is often hidden in hundreds of food products and medications. (We'll discuss how to spot hidden lactose in Chapter Four.)

After one to two weeks on this less-restricted diet, if your symptoms disappear, you're most likely lactose intolerant. But, even if you're symptoms DON'T go away, you STILL may be lactose intolerant. If you accidently consumed lactose—even though you were trying hard to avoid it—your self-test will be inconclusive.

If your particular case is hard to diagnose, consider seeing a doctor. He or she can prescribe medical tests to determine lactose intolerance.

Before you take these tests, your doctor probably will ask you to take the one- to two-week dairy elimination test first. So, if you've avoided it up until this point, it's better to get it over with. Then, he or she will use one or more tests to confirm the diagnosis.

There are two main tests:

Hydrogen Breath test

The hydrogen breath test is the preferred and most common method. It measures the amount of hydrogen in the air you breathe out. The test is pretty simple and noninvasive. This test is done at an outpatient clinic or doctor's office. Before the test, you'll be asked to do a selective fast. (Your doctor will tell you what not to eat or drink before the test.)

When the testing begins, you'll be instructed to breathe into a balloon-type container. Next, you'll be asked to drink a flavored liquid containing lactose. Then, over a period of hours, samples of your breathe will be collected again, and your hydrogen levels will be measured. Normally very little hydrogen should be present in your system so, if the test results show you have low levels of hydrogen, you DON'T have lactose intolerance.

But if your body has trouble breaking down and absorbing lactose, your breath hydrogen levels will increase. If your hydrogen levels are high, it's likely you have lactose intolerance. If your doctor isn't satisfied with the results, he or she might order more tests.

Note: The hydrogen breath test is generally reserved for older children and adults. It's not performed on infants because the testing technique (the use of a lactose-filled fluid and selective fasting) can lead to diarrhea in infants.

Lactose tolerance blood test

The lactose tolerance blood test looks for glucose in your blood because your body creates glucose when lactose breaks down.

For this test, you won't be allowed to eat or drink anything after midnight. After your overnight fast, you'll get a lactose-filled liquid to drink. Then blood samples are taken over two hours to measure your blood sugar levels.

After you drink the lactose solution, if you don't have lactose intolerance, you'll be able to digest the lactose drink and your blood sugar level will increase considerably. But, if you're lactose intolerant, your blood sugar level will stay the same.

How to test for a milk allergy

As mentioned, lactose intolerance is often confused with a milk allergy. Here's a way to test for it. You should drink at least two eight-ounce glasses of milk on an empty stomach and pay attention to any intestinal symptoms that develop over the next four hours. Repeat the test again, on an empty stomach, using several ounces of HARD cheese. (Think parmesan, aged gouda, gruyere, romano, or white stilton, rather than mozzarella, munster or brie.) Hard cheeses don't contain much lactose because the majority of lactose is reduced by the fermentation process.

If you get symptoms from the milk but not the cheese, you're probably lactose intolerant. If symptoms occur with both milk and cheese, you may be allergic to dairy products.

Be aware

An allergy to milk is *much more serious* than intolerance to lactose. If you are allergic to milk, talk to your doctor. Eating dairy with a milk allergy increases the risk of anaphylaxis—a rare but serious allergic reaction that happens rapidly and may cause death.

Don't mess around with this stuff

While a milk allergy can be dangerous, severe lactose intolerance can also be a serious health problem. The inability to digest and absorb lactose irritates the lining of the intestines. This irritation leads to a weakened digestive system that exposes you to future systemic (affecting your entire body) disorders.

In addition to an inability to absorb needed nutrients, a weakened digestive system is more susceptible to attack by parasites, yeast and pathogenic bacteria (bacteria that cause infection) which only worsens the problems in your intestines and exposes you to chronic disease.

If you're both lactose intolerant and allergic to dairy, you could face even more health consequences

What if it's NOT lactose intolerance or a dairy allergy? If your symptoms persist even after you stop dairy and lactose, you may have developed a more serious condition that needs to be treated.

There are a number of other conditions that mimic the symptoms of lactose intolerance but, because the areas affected in the gastrointestinal tract (GI tract) are different, the essential treatments for these conditions are different.

Here's a partial list:

Celiac disease

Celiac disease is an autoimmune condition where the body's immune system starts attacking normal tissue, such as intestinal tissue, in response to eating gluten.

Crohn's disease

Crohn's disease is a chronic inflammatory condition of the gastrointestinal tract; it's one of a group of diseases called inflammatory bowel disease (IBD) that causes inflammation of the lining of the digestive system.

Ulcerative colitis

Ulcerative colitis is also an inflammatory bowel disease that causes ulcers in the lining of the rectum and colon. Ulcers form where inflammation has killed the cells that usually line the colon.

Don't guess

You need to be sure why you're experiencing symptoms. If you have only one takeaway from this book, I want this to be it:

Be aware and check with your doctor. Your good health, I believe, should be your highest priority.

Chapter Three
Why Me?

I'll admit it; sometimes in the past I felt pretty sorry for myself. Ending up at an ice cream parlor with a bunch of my friends and watching then eat bowlfuls of ice cream, while I went without, could put me in a pretty bad mood. Why was I being singled out?

When I found out just how common lactose intolerance is, I started to feel a little better. I wasn't the only one—and neither are you.

You are not alone

You may be surprised to learn that some form of lactose intolerance affects up to **seventy-five percent** of the world's population.

According to researchers, there are some groups of people who are more likely to experience symptoms than others. Lactose intolerance is especially widespread among people of African, Asian, Native American, Mexican and

Mediterranean ancestry. Within these groups of people, sixty to ninety percent of them will be lactose intolerant to one degree or another.

Other races and ethnic groups suffer less because they tend to generate more lactase. For example, only ten to fifteen percent of people of Northern or Western European ancestry are affected by lactose intolerance.

Here's the breakdown

Note: Not everyone in these groups who has lactose intolerance will experience full-blown symptoms.

97-100	percent of African Blacks
90-100	percent of Asians
70-75	percent of North American Blacks
70-80	percent of Mexicans
60-90	percent of Mediterranean ancestry
60-80	percent of Jewish descent
10-12	percent of Middle Europeans
7-15	percent of North American Caucasians
1-5	percent of Northern Europeans

So why do some races and ethnic groups develop lactose intolerance while others don't? Researchers from Cornell University believe that it has to do with each group's environment and how they adapted to it.

For example, ethnic groups whose ancestors came from climates that had the right conditions for dairy cattle, like Europe, can digest milk better than those from places that didn't have the right conditions for raising dairy cattle—like Asia and Africa.

All in all, an estimated fifty million Americans are lactose intolerant.

Some reasons why you could be lactose intolerant:

Your genes

As you can see, there's a genetic component to lactose intolerance. For example, if you come from a group of people that tends to have more lactose intolerance, chances are you'll have a greater chance of developing it. If a member of your family is lactose intolerant, the probability increases.

Surgery or trauma

While age and genetics are the strongest indicators of who will develop this condition, injuries to the small intestine (surgery or trauma) can also increase your risk for developing lactose intolerance. If your small intestine is injured, most likely this condition will be temporary. Your intestines will begin producing lactase again after the intestine has healed.

But, in some cases, it could be permanent. In this case, the intestines will simply no longer be able to produce the lactase that's needed to break down the lactose.

Stomach flu

Have you suffered from the stomach flu? Sometimes people who suffer from regular bouts of the flu might also suffer from lactose intolerance, but it's usually temporary and goes away as soon as the flu does.

People experience lactose intolerance in different ways.

How about you?

Symptoms of lactose intolerance can vary depending on the severity of the intolerance. Symptoms can range from uncomfortable, but harmless, bloating to severe cramping and diarrhea. If you have severe lactose intolerance, you may experience symptoms of lactose intolerance within a half hour of eating or drinking foods with lactose. If your lactose intolerance is mild or moderate, it may take two hours until you notice symptoms. Not everyone has the same reaction; it usually varies a bit from individual to individual. In general, there are two categories of people who are lactose intolerant:

Group One: People with mild to moderate lactose intolerance

This first group can handle small amounts of lactose and, by making just a few changes in their diet, they can reduce the symptoms. If you're in Group One, you may be able to drink a glass of milk each day and eat dairy products like butter and cheese on a regular basis.

Group Two: People with severe lactose intolerance

The second group is made up of people who can't digest *any* amount of lactose. If your body has completely stopped producing lactase, you may develop extreme reactions to even the tiniest amounts of lactose—like I did. If you're in this group, you'll need to make a dramatic shift to a lactose-free lifestyle if you want to be free of your symptoms.

I know this may sound difficult, but I did it and I know you can, too. You'll learn much more about strategies for overcoming severe lactose intolerance in Chapter Five.

Chapter Four
Mild to Moderate Lactose Intolerance

If you're experiencing mild to moderate lactose intolerance symptoms, you know it can be difficult and bothersome to live with. Where you are along the spectrum of lactose intolerance will determine what dietary changes you need to make. With mild to moderate lactose intolerance symptoms, you'll have a lot more flexibility in your diet and much fewer restrictions.

How to manage your mild to moderate lactose intolerance

By experimenting, most people with mild to moderate lactose intolerance discover they can still eat small amounts of dairy and other foods containing lactose without triggering symptoms such as bloating, gas, abdominal discomfort, diarrhea or nausea. The key is to keep track of how much lactose you eat and what you can tolerate.

How much is not too much?

As a rule of thumb, people who have mild to moderate lactose intolerance can generally digest an average of *ten grams* of lactose every twenty-four hours. This may be your personal benchmark, or you may find you can tolerate more.

And, surprisingly, if you keep eating these small amounts of dairy and lactose, you may be able to stimulate some additional lactase production, which, in turn, will help you better tolerate dairy products—a full circle.

The key is to know your lactose limit

You may know your symptoms pretty well by now and what you can handle. Perhaps you already keep a mental record of foods or amounts to avoid. You may also want to start jotting down notes. You can keep a food diary and note when, what and how much you ate, and how it affected you. Using a diary allows you to see patterns and get a handle on specific foods and the symptoms they cause. (In Chapter Five you'll find extensive information on setting up and keeping a food diary.)

So, how about lasagna, tomato bisque, chili cheese steak, macaroni and cheese, or fill in the blank? As you experiment with eating dairy products, you'll figure out how much your digestive system can tolerate. Were you bloated, uncomfortable, crampy, or worse? Note it in your diary. You should be able to look back and see a definite pattern emerging.

Just how much is ten grams a day?

The answer depends on which dairy foods you consume and in what quantities. You might be surprised to hear that, on ten grams a day, you could potentially butter your toast, have cream in your coffee, eat a cup of yogurt, and shake a little Parmesan onto your pasta.

Here's a quick reference for you:

Take a look at the lactose levels of the most popular dairy foods. Common baking ingredients made from dairy, including dry milk powder, sweetened condensed milk, evaporated milk, and buttermilk, all have high levels of lactose, as do ice cream and milk. At the low end of the lactose spectrum are aged cheeses, butter and margarine, which can be consumed in small quantities.

The lactose list:

- Nonfat dry milk powder, 1 cup: 62 grams of lactose

- Sweetened condensed milk, 1 cup: 40 grams of lactose

- Evaporated milk, 1 cup: 24 grams of lactose

- Milk (nonfat, 1%, 2%, whole), 1 cup: 11 grams of lactose

- Ice cream, 1 cup: 12 grams of lactose

- Buttermilk, 1 cup: 10 grams of lactose

- Yogurt, low fat, 1 cup: 5 grams of lactose

- Sherbet, orange, ½ cup: 4 grams of lactose

- Half and half, ½ cup: 5 grams of lactose

- Sour cream, ½ cup: 4 grams of lactose

- Cream, light, ½ cup: 4 grams of lactose

- Whipping cream, ½ cup: 3 grams of lactose

- Cottage cheese, creamed, ½ cup: 3 grams of lactose

- Cottage cheese, un-creamed, ½ cup: 2 grams of lactose

- Cream cheese, 1 ounce: 1 gram of lactose

- Hard cheeses (like parmesan, romano, white stilton):
  1 ounce: 0-1 gram of lactose
- Butter, 1 tsp.: trace amounts of lactose
- Margarine, 1 tsp.: trace amounts of lactose

Hidden in plain sight

In addition to dairy products, many prepared and processed foods on supermarket shelves—from baking mixes to salad dressings—contain dairy products. Manufacturers don't always list lactose as one of their ingredients. To be safe, check labels for "hidden" lactose that comes from ingredients such as: butter, casein, cheese, cream, curds, milk, milk by-products, milk solids, milk sugar, dry milk products, non-fat dry milk powder, whey, nougat and yogurt. Also avoid items that state "may contain milk" on the food label.

Other foods that may contain lactose in smaller quantities include:

- Bread and baked goods

- Milk chocolate

- Sauces

- Breakfast cereals and cereal bars

- Instant foods such as breakfast drink mixes, mashed potatoes, soups, rice and noodle mixes

- Processed meats like bacon, hot dogs, sausage and lunch meats (other than kosher). See Chapter Five for more information about kosher foods.

- Candies and other snacks

- Mixes for pancakes, biscuits, and cookies

- Margarine

- Organ meats (such as liver)

- Sugar beets, peas, lima beans

So how much can you eat?

If you're not sure which lactose-containing foods you can handle, experiment with one dairy food at a time. You should be able to tell whether the food bothers you within thirty minutes to two hours after eating it. For example, eat a half-cup of cottage cheese and see how well you tolerate it.

If you don't have symptoms from the food and amount you try, slowly keep increasing the amount to see at what point you do have symptoms. For instance, you may find you don't have symptoms with a half-cup of cottage cheese, but you do with a cup. So your tolerance level is probably three-quarters of a cup. Keep track.

If you do have symptoms, try cutting back on the amount to see if you can handle a smaller portion.

Maybe you can't enjoy a big glass of milk with a slice of your favorite chocolate cake, but you can try a smaller serving. Start with a four-ounce glass instead of a full eight-ounce one. Gradually increase the amount of dairy you eat until you begin to notice those all-to-familiar unpleasant symptoms. Listen to your body; you'll know when you've reached your limit.

Important: if you want to eat more than this, give your stomach at least an hour or two to digest the first serving. This will help to prevent symptoms from developing.

Once you've found how much of one food you can tolerate, start testing another food. Don't try to test multiple dairy and lactose products at the same time. It's too confusing.

Remember you're in charge—**don't let lactose take control of your diet**. Here are some suggestions:

Put dairy on the side

Instead of just eating or drinking dairy products, like milk or ice cream, on their own, try having them with other nondairy foods.

For some people, combining dairy with other foods to create a whole meal may reduce or even eliminate their usual symptoms. So don't just drink a glass of milk in the morning; pour it over your cereal or oatmeal and have a piece of toast on the side, or perhaps add an egg to the meal.

Choose cheese wisely

Yes, you can still eat cheese if you have mild to moderate lactose intolerance, but choose wisely. Hard, aged cheeses like parmesan, aged gouda, romano and white stilton are lower in lactose. Other lower-lactose cheese options include provolone and munster. Certain types of cheeses—especially soft cheeses like mozzarella, or creamy ones like brie—are higher in lactose. Make a list of all the potential low-lactose cheeses you can eat; bring it to the grocery store and experiment. You may find you like many of these low-lactose cheeses, making it possible to add more variety to your diet.

Coffee creamers

A lot of people are hooked on convenient coffee creamers. If you're one of them, the good news is that you'll find a wide variety of **non-dairy** creamers on the market. You might discover that you like these creamers even better than dairy-filled ones, or even milk, in your coffee.

But, be aware that some non-dairy creamers have trace amounts of lactose and are often high in fat compared to creamers made from cow's milk. Be sure to consider this if you add non-dairy creamers to your diet. Don't confuse non-dairy with fat-free or low-fat. Look at all the available brands and choose the healthiest.

Coffee creamers can be expensive. Membership stores like Costco and Sam's often offer large cases of creamers that can bring the price per individual creamer way down. If you can't use all the creamers before the expiration date, perhaps you can find someone to share with.

Other options: reduced lactose

Choose reduced-lactose products. Reduced-lactose products taste, for the most part, like regular dairy products, but the lactose—the natural sugar content—has been modified or reduced for people who are lactose intolerant.

If you find you're experiencing symptoms with reduced-lactose products, you may want to go all the way and try totally lactose-free and dairy-free choices. You'll find there are almost always alternatives to any lactose choice. Decide which items you're willing to give up and go for their alternatives.

Milk alternatives

One suggestion: try eliminating your biggest source of daily lactose first. For most people it's fresh milk. If you want to avoid lactose completely, in addition to using lactose-free dairy milk, try non-dairy beverages like soy milk (my favorite). Soy is a great source of protein and a variety of micronutrients.

But you don't have to stick with soy. There are many other milk-alternative beverages you can try. You'll find almond, rice and coconut milk in most grocery stores. Many of the varieties have a chocolate version, which gives you even more options. Check out health food stores for less well-known choices like oat, cashew nut, and hemp milk. You might like almond milk in your coffee and coconut milk on your cereal. Don't be afraid to experiment.

It may take you some time to get used to these alternative tastes. It took me a few days to get used to the taste of soy in my coffee; now I wouldn't have it any other way.

But be careful as you try these new products. Some people may find they have an intolerance to one or more of these milk alternatives. Again, here's where your food diary will come in handy to help you determine the cause of any digestive stress.

Nutritional supplements

Many canned nutritional supplements (such as Ensure) are lactose-free. Check the product labels.

Ask the professionals

I know learning a new way of eating isn't easy, but perhaps you may not have to do it alone. Ask your doctor to recommend a nutritionist or dietitian to help you manage your diet. He or she can teach you how to read food labels, share healthy eating tips, determine how much dairy you can tolerate without symptoms, and come up with reduced-lactose or lactose-free alternatives to provide a well-balanced diet.

The nutritionist I talked to recommended a powdered protein shake that's classified as a medical food. It contains no wheat, gluten, corn protein, yeast, animal, *dairy* products, fish, shellfish, peanuts, tree nuts, egg, artificial colors, artificial sweeteners, or preservatives. It also contains the supplement glutamine to help heal the gut. The product is called "OptiCleanse GHI made by Xymogen. (I have no connection with Xymogen and I don't receive any monetary compensation. I only offer this product as something that works for me.) You can find it on the Internet.

I add soy milk to one of these shakes every morning for breakfast. It's a great alternative to sometimes struggling to find lactose-free breakfast items. I like eggs—but not all the time. I even make a second shake for lunch some days if I'm extra busy.

Note: Many people develop a food intolerance to soy over time. Be aware of this if you notice any symptoms while drinking soy milk.

I know that meeting with a nutritionist or dietitian can be expensive, especially if it's not covered by your health insurance. If this resource isn't available to you, you can accomplish everything you need to do yourself. Take some time, educate yourself and put together a detailed plan. Let this be your guide for overcoming your symptoms and for healthy living.

Got lactase supplements?

It's not a cure, but taking lactase enzyme supplements (you can find them in most drug stores and health food stores) can help you tolerate foods containing lactose. If you use a supplement, you even may be able to eat heavy cream dishes and ice cream without symptoms. And, if you don't know the exact ingredients of any dish you're eating, you can protect yourself from hidden lactose by taking a lactase supplement before eating a "mystery meal."

You can find supplements in a variety of forms including liquid, caplets, and chewable tablets. Read the labels of these products carefully because they all work differently. Some have to be taken a day before you drink or eat dairy products. Others have to be added to your dairy products before you eat or drink them. Still others you pop in your mouth with your first bite-full of dairy.

If you don't find a kind that works for you, keep trying. I all but gave up, but after much trial and error, I was able to find two brands in a health food store that worked for me. These weren't the most popular or the best marketed; in fact, I'd never heard of one of the brands before, but they became lifesavers in my lactose-free journey.

Probiotics for lactose intolerance

You can also try probiotic supplements. For some people, probiotics can help with digestion and ease symptoms of lactose intolerance. I found my symptoms improved when I started taking them.

Probiotics are live microorganisms, usually bacteria, which restore the balance of "good" bacteria in the digestive system by pushing the "bad" bacteria out. With more than four hundred species of bacteria living inside our intestines, it's essential that we keep the levels of good and bad bacteria in balance.

If you're using a supplement, be aware of the amount of live bacteria in the supplement. Each dose should be a fifty to eighty billion culture count. Buy probiotics that are in refrigerated cases (heat can kill the live bacteria). If you need more information, ask someone at a health food store or talk to a nutritionist.

Other sources of probiotics

Probiotics can be found naturally in foods like kefir and yogurt. You may not be familiar with kefir (pronounced key-fur). It's a cultured probiotic beverage similar in taste and texture to drinkable yogurt. It's made from milk fermented with kefir cultures. (The kefir grain, with its fermenting yeasts and bacteria, is added to fresh milk, which is then permitted to sour.)

The process of making kefir is more than 2000 years old. It began in the Caucasus Mountains (near Turkey) where many people live to well over one hundred years. Kefir has been associated with a long list of health benefits and is considered one of the best milk products for people suffering from lactose intolerance.

How does kefir help?

A study in the Journal of the American Dietetic Association examined people struggling with lactose intolerance and found that kefir can actually improve lactose digestion. The reasoning? Kefir's live, active bacteria cultures release enzymes that digest lactose. Both kefir and yogurt work the same way.

Good yogurt, bad yogurt?

Be careful about the yogurt products you choose.

Like kefir, yogurt can be a great food full of probiotics that can help to lessen the inflammation in the GI tract and the symptoms of lactose intolerance. And, I think yogurt is a real convenience when you need to eat something on the run.

But not all yogurts are the same. The lactose content in some yogurts can cause lactose intolerance symptoms ranging from mild to severe. If you can't find a good yogurt that doesn't trigger your symptoms, there are other options.

One solution:

Stop eating *pasteurized* yogurt. Pasteurized yogurt contains beneficial bacteria, but there's a possibility that all of the good bacteria in the yogurt is already dead due to the introduction of heat. So instead of actually being beneficial, the yogurt becomes another trigger for your lactose intolerance. (This was the case for me.)

Instead, if you can find it, choose *unpasteurized* yogurt that contains live probiotic bacteria and reap the benefits.

When this type of yogurt enters the intestines, the bacterial cultures convert lactose to lactic acid, so the yogurt will have a lower lactose content than yogurt without live cultures.

The major brands are pasteurized, so look for brands that say organic as a start, and then read the label. I checked major supermarket chains and found they don't carry any brands of unpasteurized yogurt. You may find some choices in some health food stores. But it may require some researching on your part to find those stores in your area that carry the unpasteurized version. Mountain High is a brand you can find in the West Coast markets, and Stonyfield can be found in some markets as well.

Do it yourself

An even better option is to make your own homemade yogurt. The process starts with freeze-dried bacteria available from stores like Whole Foods and Amazon. One brand is Yogourmet.

One of the benefits of making your own yogurt is you're better able to control heat settings to preserve the beneficial bacteria. You can make yogurt by hand or use a yogurt maker; there are several models available. Another benefit? It costs far less to make yogurt than to buy it.

The best yogurt solution

Did you know you can also culture nondairy milks such as almond or coconut? This way you'll get both the benefits of the good bacteria and none of the risks of lactose intolerance. An elegant solution.

Food Strategies: What to eat when you're eating out

You may have found it difficult to eat at restaurants in the past without having your symptoms flair. But now, if you follow the guidelines in this book, you should be able to eat at restaurants without too much fuss. It may take a little detective work on your part.

To begin, be sure to ask your server if dishes are made with butter, milk or cheese or, if your server isn't sure, ask the chef to come to your table. I've found that chefs, for the most part, seem very happy to oblige.

You should be able to spot non lactose-laden food choices like salads (without cheese) and meats and fish on your own. Just be wary of already-buttered bread (those wonderful hot loaves they bring to the table), salad dressings and creamy sauces and cheeses.

Indian restaurants can be particularly good choices. They offer curry dishes, chicken dishes and delicious, crunchy bread made without dairy—all foods that likely won't trigger lactose intolerance symptoms.

The majority of Asian cooking is made without dairy. Try sushi or other Japanese dishes; look for Thai and Vietnamese delicacies. If you've never eaten Asian dishes before, this may be a great opportunity to expand your palate. You may be surprised at how delicious Asian cooking can be. And Mediterranean-style cooking, for the most part, is made without dairy products. Check out Italian and Spanish restaurants. (For more extensive dining-out tips, see Chapter Five.)

Fast food

We all know that most fast food is not a healthy choice but, sometimes, you just don't have a choice. If you need to go that way, be educated. Most chains will provide their nutritional information at their store locations or online. With this information, you can make informed choices. I pulled these items off internet sites to give you an idea. Note: these are in milligrams, not grams. There are 1000 milligrams in one gram.

McDonald's

Big Mac (without Big Mac sauce)

Lactose = 350mg

Quarter Pounder

Lactose = 70mg

Kentucky Fried Chicken

Biscuit

Lactose = 5000 mg

Cinnamon rolls

Lactose = 4500 mg

Burger King

Vanilla shake

Lactose = 4260mg

Eye-opening

Can you believe how much lactose there is in some of this stuff? Obviously, with these choices, you'd want to go for the Quarter Pounder at 70 mg of lactose if you could.

Use the research options available to plan your fast-food runs. If you're prepared, you don't have to fall off the wagon and suffer the consequences. If you know in advance which lactose-free items you can order at several of the chains, you'll be able to make an informed decision and still eat on the run.

(See Chapter Five for more information on making wise choices when ordering fast food.)

Dinner parties

You have a little more flexibility when eating with friends. Most people understand dietary restrictions. Just let your host know in advance that you need to eat limited lactose. Ask what's on the menu and, if need be, bring something you can eat that compliments the meal.

Your host may even be kind enough to offer to cook an entire lactose-free meal that works for everyone. If you want, you can bring additional items to share that you know you can tolerate. (A side dish or a non-dairy dessert perhaps?) See the recipes in PART TWO for ideas.

Take a lactase supplement

I always keep lactase supplements with me because I never know when I'll need them. I personally recommend taking a supplement at the beginning of a dinner party because dairy products can often slip in unnoticed. And to increase your odds of a non-symptom meal, eat simply.

Stay away from sour cream, cream sauces, soft cheeses and dairy desserts.

Just gotta have some dairy? Make a decision. If you can handle it, decide which dairy products you most want to eat and then choose wisely. Want the crème brulee? Forgo the cream-based sauces and the mozzarella appetizers. Want the lasagna? Eliminate the ice cream. It's a balancing act but, if you're careful, you can have your entree and your dessert, too. Your food diary can be a big help in making good choices.

Chapter 5
Living with Severe Lactose Intolerance

The lactose-free lifestyle

You'll find some of the information, tips and techniques from Chapter Four repeated here in Chapter Five. But, while some of the steps in the previous chapter may be optional for people with mild to moderate lactose intolerance, if you have severe lactose intolerance, you'll need to follow each one carefully and completely.

But the good news is that, although severe lactose intolerance can affect your health and perhaps your quality of life, it's not life threatening AND you can reduce or eliminate your symptoms. While there's no drug that will cure it—there can be a dietary cure.

The cure for severe lactose intolerance is to completely eliminate lactose from your diet. Period.

When you stop consuming lactose, your painful and sometimes embarrassing symptoms will disappear, and your digestive issues will heal. To those with the most difficult and severe symptoms, it probably will seem like a small price to pay.

In order to go lactose-free, you'll need to make sweeping changes in your lifestyle. You'll have to be motivated enough to change your daily eating habits even though these habits are powerful and, most likely, hard to break. If you want to shift to a lactose-free lifestyle, you'll have to replace your ingrained habits with healthier choices. But please don't feel overwhelmed. The solution is to make these lifestyle changes in a slow and controlled manner.

First of all, you'll need some time to learn about all the food products that have lactose in them and to look for lactose-free substitutes. Once you have this knowledge and a few lactose-free items in your pantry, you can begin planning for your lactose-free lifestyle. Remember, you don't have to do this overnight. Start out gradually and ease yourself into this healthy new lifestyle.

Getting started

You'll find a good deal of information here that will help you as you eliminate all sources of lactose in your diet and move into this new, lactose-free way of living—a lifestyle that will support your health, well-being and peace of mind.

You CAN do it

First and foremost, pat yourself on the back for making a healthy move away from dairy products and lactose-filled foods. Of course, let's face it—milk, cream, ice cream and other dairy products are tasty—okay, fabulous.

But sometimes tasting good isn't enough. Severe stomach cramping and pain can outweigh any pleasure from eating these offending foods. I know it did for me. It's really pointless to continue to eat food products that taste good but cause you such pain and—if you need more incentive—it's also unhealthy.

But the good news is there are dozens upon dozens of products on the market that taste good, are good for you, and won't cause you any intestinal problems.

Yes, you can achieve your ultimate goal—to be free of the unwelcome symptoms of lactose intolerance.

Note: If you don't have lactose intolerance, but you still want to shift to a lactose-free lifestyle for health or other reasons, of course that's alright, too. For example, vegans choose to eliminate dairy products from their diet along with meat, fish and poultry.

The challenges of the lactose-free lifestyle

You'll face several challenges when you decide to move to a lactose-free lifestyle. The two biggest:

1. Learning to avoid products that have hidden lactose

2. Discovering how to eat and drink the right dairy substitutes and various whole foods so you can stay healthy and get the right nutrients in the right doses

Where is lactose found? You name it

Switching to a lactose-free diet is tough because lactose is everywhere. Milk is often added to many dishes we eat, and dairy products, in some form, are found in many recipes.

But there's more to consider than just dairy. Lactose is found in a wide range of prepared and processed foods. Many of these foods make up a good part of an average American's daily diet. And there are other places to look, too.

Lactose in medications? Really?

I was surprised to learn that lactose is often used as a filer or coating in some medications and many types of birth control pills. In fact, it's the base for more than twenty percent of prescription drugs and about six percent of over-the-counter medications.

Why do manufacturers do this? There are four main reasons:

1. Lactose is an almost tasteless except for a slight sweetness, making it an ideal filler.

2. Lactose prevents caking for chewable-type tablets

3. Lactose can be sprayed onto a pill to product a shiny, hard coating, making pills easier to swallow.

4. Hardly anybody is bothered by small amounts of lactose.

"Hardly anybody" isn't much comfort if you're one of those sufferers. If you are extremely sensitive and can't tolerate any lactase in your system, you could possibly have a reaction to the medications you're taking. Pills containing lactose are obviously not compatible with a lactose-free lifestyle

What to do? First of all you shouldn't be alarmed. There are alternatives to every pill. Every type of medication has at least one lactose-free variety or manufacturer. Both physicians and pharmacists will have the latest edition of the Physicians' Desk Reference (PDR). This reference book lists all inactive ingredients in virtually all prescription medications.

Probably the best course of action when you drop off your prescription is to ask your pharmacist to research your drug to see if it contains lactose. This will give him or her a chance to find an equivalent drug for you, if necessary.

Over–the-counter medications

Non-prescription drugs or "(over-the-counter (OTC)" medications are easier to research. Luckily, virtually all companies list their inactive ingredients on the sides of their packages and often on their websites. You'll also find that many brands of vitamins and minerals do the same.

You should be able to find a lactose-free alternative that meets your needs.

Foods you should avoid

If you're striving for a lactose-free diet, again you'll need to eliminate *all* dairy. Here's a list to make sure you're targeting the most commonly used products.

Note: This list is repeated from Chapter Four, which contains strategies for people with mild to moderate lactose intolerance.

But now this information becomes crucial if you have severe lactose intolerance.

You should avoid all of these items, except perhaps the hard cheeses, butter and margarine, which have very little lactose. You'll know what's right for your body. If you find yourself reacting to even these lowest levels of lactose, eliminate them all.

- Nonfat dry milk powder, 1 cup: 62 grams of lactose

- Sweetened condensed milk, 1 cup: 40 grams of lactose

- Evaporated milk, 1 cup: 24 grams of lactose

- Milk (nonfat, 1%, 2%, whole), 1 cup: 11 grams of lactose

- Ice cream, 1 cup: 12 grams of lactose

- Buttermilk, 1 cup: 10 grams of lactose

- Yogurt, low fat, 1 cup: 5 grams of lactose

- Sherbet, orange: ½ cup: 4 grams of lactose

- Half and half, ½ cup: 5 grams of lactose

- Sour cream, ½ cup: 4 grams of lactose

- Cream, light, ½ cup: 4 grams of lactose

- Whipping cream, ½ cup: 3 grams of lactose

- Cottage cheese, creamed, ½ cup: 3 grams of lactose

- Cottage cheese, un-creamed, ½ cup: 2 grams of lactose

- Cream cheese, 1 ounce: 1 gram of lactose

- Hard cheeses: like parmesan, romano, white stilton: 1 ounce: 0-1 gram of lactose

- Butter, 1 tsp.: trace amounts of lactose

- Margarine, 1 tsp.: trace amounts of lactose

Know what you're getting—other names for lactose

As we learned in Chapter Four, in addition to the dairy products listed here, many prepared and processed foods on supermarket shelves—from baking mixes to salad dressings—contain dairy products. Manufacturers don't always put "lactose" on the label.

To be sure, check food labels for "hidden" lactose that comes from ingredients such as butter, casein, cheese, cream, curds, milk, milk by-products, milk solids, milk sugar, dry milk products, non-fat dry milk powder, whey, nougat and yogurt. Also avoid items that state "may contain milk" on the food label.

Here's the list, once again, of other foods that may contain lactose in smaller quantities:

- Bread and baked goods

- Milk chocolate

- Mixes for waffles, pancakes, cookies and biscuits and already prepared waffles, pancakes, cookies and biscuits

- Processed breakfast foods like toaster pastries and doughnuts

- Instant foods: breakfast drink mixes, mashed potatoes, soups, rice and noodle mixes

- Processed meats like bacon, hot dogs, sausage and lunch meats (other than kosher). More information on kosher foods follows.

- Sauces

- Margarine

- Non-dairy whipped toppings

- Nondairy creamers (liquid and powdered—contain only trace amounts)

- Processed snacks like potato chips and corn chips

- Meal replacement powders and shakes

- Processed breakfast cereals and cereal bars

- Certain types of candy, such as milk chocolate

- Granola bars

- Organ meats (such as liver)

- Sugar beets, peas, lima beans

Use a Food Diary to keep you on track

You've probably head of a conventional food diary. It's a detailed record of the food and drink you consume over a given period of time—for example: one day, one week or one month. Recorded items may include the number of calories in your food, the time of day you ate, and your level of hunger when you ate. It may also contain information that tracts the amount of exercise you do. A food journal is commonly used to identify eating patterns, track calories, and to identify changes that you can make.

While this can be an excellent tool for people who want to lose weight, you can use the same principals to help you overcome your lactose intolerance. You can keep track of the food you eat, discover which foods trigger your symptoms and note the severity of your symptoms.

You'll need to include enough details in your description to help in your analysis.

Include:

- Type of food

- Brand name, if applicable

- Amount eaten: by cup, tablespoon or teaspoon, or other standard measurement

- By size, giving dimensions (length, width, thickness, or diameter)

- By number, for standard-size items

- By weight

Examples:

Cereal: Size of servings; brand name; additions such as *milk or milk substitute*, instant or ready-to-eat type?

Baked Goods: Homemade or commercial? From scratch or mix? Brand? Topping or frosting? Dimensions? Weight or number eaten?

Milk Products: Note regular milk, reduced lactose, or milk substitutions such as soy or almond.

Mixed Dishes: Homemade or commercial? From scratch or mix? Brand? Major ingredients and proportions? Cooking method?

Soups: Homemade or commercial? Brand? Broth or milk base? Type of milk? Principal ingredients?

Butter or butter substitutes: stick, tub, diet, whipped, squeeze, or liquid margarine, Brand?

Commercial salad dressing: Brand? Low calorie? Creamy? Additions?

Snacks: Brand, size, weight or number eaten?

Restaurant Meals—type: fast food, ethnic, deli, family style?

Beside each entry, you'll want to record the time you ate each item. If you experience symptoms, go back and record the type of symptoms, and rate them from mild to severe. Then record how long it took for the symptoms to occur. This will be incredibly useful information as you go forward with your lactose-free lifestyle

Getting help

While this may sound complicated, there are tools available to help you. Free food journal forms and log books are available online. (In most cases, though, you'll be asked to sign up at a website.) These websites usually offer forms that have spaces to customize your diary so you can track your lactose intolerance. Some are even made for specific conditions, such as Irritable Bowel Syndrome, which can easily be converted to track your symptoms.

Another option is to go the paid route—you can check out a variety of websites and programs.

If you don't want to go this route, you can make your own food diary using an Excel spreadsheet or similar form. Or, keep a handwritten diary or create a Word document.

It doesn't have to be anything intricate, just user friendly. Otherwise you're bound to get frustrated and give up.

Apps for tracking symptoms

Probably the easiest way to keep a food diary is to use one of the various apps made for smart phones.

Note: I haven't tried these apps myself, so I'm not able to make a recommendation. I have no monetary interest in these products and provide this information only as potential additional resources for you.

Having said this, you may want to check out "mySymptoms" by SkyGazer Labs Ltd. At the time of this book's publication, the cost for mySymptoms is $2.99.

According to the publisher, mySymptoms is a food and symptom diary that aims to provide insights into the possible triggers of your symptoms. The publisher says:

mySymptoms can be used for recording, tracking, and analyzing symptoms associated with IBS (irritable bowel syndrome), food intolerance, heartburn, Crohn's disease, eczema, asthma, allergies, diarrhea, vomiting, nausea, headaches, bloating, or any other symptom you wish to record.

You simply record your foods, drinks, medications, energy, sleep quality, stress, exercise, environmental factors, bowel movements, and any symptoms you experience to discover insights into the possible triggers of your symptoms. The more diary events you record, the more effective the analysis becomes.

You also have the option to provide your doctor or dietician with a clear view of your diet and symptoms plus additional factors such as medications, stress, exercise, etc. by generating a report of your diary for printing or sharing by email.

You can also use mySymptoms to aid your analysis during an elimination diet. (Always consult a licensed health professional prior to modifying your diet.)

The disclaimer from SkyGazer Labs Ltd:

Please note that the analysis tool uses statistical methods to identify suspect triggers and does not understand your diet or specific health circumstances. It isn't a silver bullet - it is aimed at providing insights into possible triggers to help you and your doctor/dietician as part of a broader, holistic investigation.

Other rather extensive information from the publisher, SkyGazer Labs Ltd:

DIARY

Record food, drink, medication, stress, exercise, environmental factors, and other activity and notes

Record any symptoms you experience (including intensity, duration, and notes)

Record your energy, sleep quality, and bowel movements (using Bristol scale)

View and modify your diary entries

Create and modify your own symptoms

Export your food diary as a HTML report for printing or sharing

ORGANIZER

Add or modify your own drinks, foods, medications, exercises, and other activities

Add or modify meals with your own ingredients

Add or modify detailed ingredients to any item – food, drink or medication

ANALYSIS

Analyze your food diary to see what might possibly be triggering your symptoms

The analysis window can be set between one and seventy-two hours

Optionally set the date range to analyze

Results show a list of possible suspects for a selected symptom

Detailed results for each suspect includes more specific information, a histogram and trend chart

mySymptoms includes a small database of foods, medications, exercises, and environmental factors to help get you going. If you can't find something, simply type its name in and tap the add button - it's that simple! Once added, it's conveniently there for future use. You can also create personalized meals containing the ingredients that you use, and once you've added a meal or food item, you can use it repeatedly.

Food Allergy Detective

You may also want to check out the "Food Allergy Detective." Again, I haven't used this app, so I'm not giving a recommendation.

The publisher is Evil Timmy, LLC. (Yes, I double-checked.) At the time of publication the cost is for this app is $3.99.

According to the publisher:

The app is easy to use; you just tap on what you've eaten and then later on tap if you've had any symptoms.

It can track symptoms even hours afterwards, and these can be anything from abdominal pain to headaches. You don't even need to put in what is in the foods you are eating as the app recognizes what ingredients are present and logs it all. You then have access to a graph which will grade your reactions from mild to serious. The app analyzes all the information to see if any patterns emerge to more fully recognize any food sensitivity or allergies.

This review is from appadvice.com:

http://appadvice.com/appnn/2011/05/enter-data-body-tells-app-pinpoint-trouble-foods

The creator of Food Allergy Detective has done his homework and been continually working to make this a great little tool. Journal your food choices quickly and keep track of how you feel afterwards. Soon, you'll have enough data entered and the app will start spitting out calculated graph results of which foods you are most likely sensitive to.

The interface is uncluttered and there are already categories in place (foods and common allergic reactions) and you can add your own food and reactions to the lists. This app does the data calculations for you so you don't have to worry about it.

I like how easy it is to enter foods consumed. Simply scroll through the list and tick the one or more foods you have consumed. If you are looking to enter foods like, "Whopper Jr." or "Taco Salad" that's not the way this app works. Instead, you enter specific ingredients you have consumed within foods such as eggs, cheese, fish, etc. Add more foods you suspect may be giving you trouble, but the app already includes the major allergen list.

After eating meals, check into the app as soon as you notice an unpleasant symptom. Check which symptom(s) you are experiencing and how long after eating you are experiencing them. This will pair up with the data you entered earlier regarding which foods you ate and will be able to calculate results.

Don't be under the guise that you will instantly know your food sensitivities on the first day you use it. The more data you have put in, the more accurate the results. So, start checking the graphs after several days of consistent use to see trends.

While this app can't take the place of a doctor, it sure can save you a lot of money by assisting you in tracking down troublesome foods. Get your diet back on track and start to feel better. Its simple interface is clean and uncluttered and it gets the job done. Customize it to meet your needs.

Remember, regardless of what type of diary you use—hand written, a Word doc, Excel spreadsheets, premade forms, going online to use a variety of websites or programs, or apps—what matters is that you keep one. The analysis that you conduct will give you great insight into your lactose intolerance and show you how you can eliminate your symptoms once and for all.

Get Ready to Go Lactose Free

In the next chapter, we'll discuss home cooking the lactose-free way. But first, some help with eating out.

Eating out

As you're committing to a lactose-free lifestyle, one of the biggest challenges you may face is eating out. As a trend, Americans eat out now more than ever. Just remember, as you rethink restaurant eating, your choices won't be limited, just shifted. Some of these suggestions will also apply to your home cooking. (See Chapter Six.)

Dairy-free dining-out tips

First—ask questions. This is by far the most important tip. Don't be afraid to ask about the ingredients of a dish, or to request changes to a menu item.

I was hesitant to do this in the past because I got a lot of, "We don't make substitutions," responses and was made to feel like I was being unreasonable. But times have changed. Today, any good waiter will be able to help, and won't hesitate to ask the chef if you want more information.

Many restaurants have caught up with new demands. People want to be able to avoid foods they're allergic or sensitive to. Low-carb devotees are demanding more low-carb selections, and dieters are requesting smaller portions. In fact, research shows that an increasing number of restaurants are providing flexibility in food preparation methods, varied portion sizes, and expanded menu offerings. They know that the key to success is to respect their customers and their specific dining needs.

Pick your restaurants wisely. Search out local restaurants that are following this trend. Local Google searches can help because they give you the opportunity to read menus thoroughly and thoughtfully in advance.

Keep Kosher to go dairy-free

Kosher food is based on the laws of the Jewish religion. The Hebrew word "kosher" means "fit or proper." Besides other dietary restrictions, Jewish law forbids the mixing of meat and milk at a meal.

People who keep kosher for religious reasons are very strict about not mixing dairy and meat. No dairy by-products of any kind are allowed into kosher stores or restaurants that serve meat.

Seek out kosher restaurants if they're available. They're usually found in areas with a high Jewish population. Delis can be a good place to start. Ask Jewish friends if they can help. Even if they don't keep kosher, they may know of kosher restaurants in your area.

Fortunately, many non-Jewish communities have also embraced the kosher dining philosophy. Some restaurants now keep kosher because so many people have embraced eating kosher for health purposes or moral reasons, such as vegetarianism.

As a part of my research for this book, I was surprised to learn that some Subway restaurants in the Unites States have gone kosher. The world's first kosher Subway restaurant opened in Cleveland. You can also find kosher Subways in Brooklyn, Kansas City and Miami. More may have opened since the publication of this book.

I found out that Subway is the world's largest submarine sandwich franchise and operates in one hundred and two countries around the world. If you have Subway restaurants in your area, you may want to check locally to see if any keep kosher.

In the United States, in my state of Florida, there are now more than one hundred different kosher restaurants according to a list compiled by Hanefesh (one of the largest database listings of kosher restaurant in the United States). You may be able to find similar organizations in other countries.

Visit websites

Once you start learning about lactose intolerance, you'll probably want to seek out more information. Websites devoted to lactose-free information are wide-ranging and can provide enormous help.

As one example, I used the Internet to find out more about kosher foods. There are many websites that share this kind of information. (See the Resources and References section.)

Forget fried foods

Fried foods are often coated with products containing lactose and laden with fat and "miscellaneous" ingredients. And of course, in addition to avoiding lactose, giving up fried foods also means a healthier lifestyle.

Look for heart-healthy oils

The menu will usually specify if a dish is cooked in oil or butter, but if in doubt, just ask. Most kitchens will have vegetable and olive oils on hand. Also, when ordering whole meats, fish, or vegetables, request that no butter is added. Some chefs automatically add a pat to grilled and steamed foods for flavor.

Dining Mediterranean style

Mediterranean cuisine features fruits and lots of vegetables and includes whole grains, olive oil, fish, nuts, beans and legumes. It typically doesn't include items that are high in saturated fats—such as butter. You can generally find several choices of Mediterranean-style food in many restaurants. When ordering pasta dishes, for example, Mediterranean style means sauces will be tomato- and olive oil-based rather than cream-based. You'll be able to avoid lactose, save yourself loads of saturated fat, and the tomato sauce can even be counted as a serving of vegetables.

Other choices for non-dairy cuisine—go ethnic

Many dairy-free patrons, in fact, eat like well-travelled food connoisseurs, even if they've never left the United States. For example, choosing African, Greek, and Italian dishes requires a bit more care, but these cuisines are also loaded with delicious dairy-free options.

As mentioned in Chapter Four, Indian and Asian restaurants are also great choices because the majority of their cooking is made without dairy. For example, Thai, Chinese, Vietnamese and Japanese are all virtually dairy free. If you've never tried many of these cuisines, be a little brave and venture out.

Look South of the Border

Mexican and Tex-Mex are still trending in the United States. Restaurants like Chipotle Mexican Grill and Tia's Tex-Mex are going strong. Items like tortillas stuffed with a mix of creations are good, and also good for on-the-go. Of course, just be sure to hold the cheese and sour cream.

Now is the time to experiment. Notice how these dishes are prepared. Many of them will probably spark some ideas for home cooking.

Soup or salad?

If you choose a salad, you'll have an excellent opportunity to get your greens, and a first-rate way to go lactose-free. Of course, just remember to order it without cheese, and choose your dressing wisely.

Go for oil & vinegar, honey mustard, French, or vinaigrettes. Avoid the heavy ranch and blue cheese choices. Mustard, ketchup, barbecue sauce, and mayonnaise are usually dairy-less, but keep it light to limit your sugar and fat intake.

On the side instead of over the top

Ask that your condiments and salad dressings come on the side. This is a very common request; in fact some restaurants no longer dress salads in the kitchen. You'll benefit from portion control and the ability to give the condiment a once over before drenching your greens.

Check on the cheese

Some chefs love to sprinkle Parmesan on just about everything. Even if you've told your server that you're ordering dairy-free, it's probably a good idea to reinforce your message. Make it simple. Just say, "And there won't be any cheese on that right?" and you've made your point twice.

Going for the soup?

Soups are a good choice if you want a heartier selection. And with many dairy-free options to choose from, you're likely to find ones you like. Many restaurants are even serving up vegan "cream" soups, which means they are meat and dairy free. Although several safe soup options may appear obvious (chicken noodle, vegetable, chili, split pea), your best option is to ask what dairy-free soups are available. You may get even more soup options in health-food restaurants. Many make their own fresh soups every day, and many are vegan.

Give meatless meals a try

Over the past few years, most restaurants have added a vegan option or two to their menus. Although most are noted as "vegetarian" (meatless), the growing trend of cutting out all animal products has turned most vegetarian dishes into vegan ones (which means, as mentioned, meat and dairy free). You may find you like going meatless once or twice a week—another healthy option.

Lighten the load for that potato

Skip the sour cream, butter, and cheese that come on a "loaded" baked potato or are whipped into mashed potatoes. Salsa, non-dairy salad dressings, or a touch of salt and pepper can add ample flavor to a baked potato. Better yet, choose roasted, steamed or boiled potatoes. Sweet potatoes are another option. I think they taste better plain than white potatoes do when all that "good stuff" is eliminated.

Substitutes for butter

Many restaurants offer fantastic dips and spreads for your bread, appetizers, and meal. Experiment with flavored oils, sweet and savory salsas, tapenades, fresh guacamole, or hummus. Keep these in mind for your kitchen, too. They're helpful to have on hand. And now, guacamole and hummus are staples in most grocery stores.

More menu methods

Selecting menu items that are baked, grilled, dry-sautéed, broiled, poached, or steamed will yield the healthiest food. You'll also have better odds of it being dairy-free. Of course, always double check that butter wasn't added, you might not be able to see it on the finished dish.

Home style—the old-fashioned way

The way you used to make it at home is probably how they're still making it at restaurant. Pancakes, waffles, scrambled eggs, and other traditional fare are typically made with a good helping of milk, so you may want to avoid them.

Watch for trending diet fads

The new diet and health options listed on many menus typically are made without cream or cheese. You not only get to go lactose-free, but lower your calories.

Take it black

Try your coffee and tea without milk and cream. You may be surprised to find you like it. If you discover it's not for you, try a dairy-free substitute. For example, ask the restaurant if they have soymilk; you'll be surprised how many places do. (Starbucks for one.) I haven't found any places that carry alternative milk options besides soy.

I once asked for soymilk for my coffee at a Barnes & Noble café, and was told they didn't provide it. But the helpful barista, seeing the disappointed look on my face, actually went in the back and brought out a whole cup of soymilk for me—no charge. (Which left me wondering why they just didn't make it available in the first place?)

It's a little less convenient, but, as a backup, you can always bring along your own packet of soy or rice-based creamer. (Check health food stores.)

Do dessert later

Craving dessert? Head home for one of your own dazzling dessert recipes (See Part Two for recipes) or store-bought treats. Restaurant desserts are typically quite heavy (translation, full of cream and butter). If you must have dessert, fruit and sorbet options are usually safe.

Fast food?

Should you really be eating fast food? Well "no" is the obvious answer, but sometimes there are no other options:

You're running to an appointment—you're late, you're hungry and your only option for sustenance is to pass through a drive thru. You're on the road traveling, trying to make a destination before dark, and you can't afford the hassle and downtime of a sit-down meal. You're at an airport, waiting for your flight, and there's nothing much to eat except fried foods, donuts, pizza or smoothies. (Thank goodness many large airports now offer better choices.)

If you find yourself trapped in a similar situation, don't give in or give up and just go for the lactose. You can survive fast food without triggering your symptoms. You just have to be diligent.

Go green

Opt for the salads without cheese. Some chains may have dressings that contain lactose. (Luckily fast-food dressings always come on the side.) Ask what lactose-free options are available, but don't expect much, you'll most likely get blank stares. Check the ingredients if you can, or go without the dressing.

If you can, look online before-hand for nutritional information and you'll know for sure which dressings to pick and which to avoid.

Eat real food

Choose the most "whole-looking" options. If it's fried and unrecognizable, it's probably in a coating with unknown ingredients—including lactose.

Pick the best

Sandwich shops and delis vary in quality. As mentioned, a kosher deli is probably the best choice but, if you're not near one, choose the highest quality you can find. The good thing about a sandwich is that it doesn't need cheese to taste good. Mayo is almost always dairy-free, but it doesn't hurt to ask for a smaller dollop anyway for the benefit of your overall health. Avoid the croissants though—there's usually enough butter in these to quickly trigger your symptoms.

Check for soups

Look for bean, tomato, vegetable, Mexican tortilla, split pea and chili. Some fast food places have daily soups, but you may have to look around. Again, check the nutritional information online, if you can, before venturing in.

Treat yourself

Seek out the "fancier" fast food restaurants. There's a growing trend now for "fast-casual" chains. They try to offer the quality foods of nicer sit-down restaurants in a fast-food atmosphere. Again, Chipotle Mexican Grill comes to mind because they source organic and local produce when practical.

Do your homework

If you scope out fast food restaurants before you venture out, you'll have a much better chance of knowing which foods you can eat. As mentioned, go online to view menus, look for lactose information and check out other items like calorie counts and food allergy lists as well.

Use good judgment

Lactose-free fast food choices are clear-cut when you can check nutritional information. Scan the menu for your best and most enticing options. It may take some trial and error, but you'll quickly learn to pick the winners.

Remember, these tips are general guidelines, but there are no dairy-free guarantees when dining out. When in doubt, ASK. Also, if you have severe food allergies in addition to lactose intolerance, you should use extra caution as cross-contamination of milk and other food allergens is highly possible in restaurant kitchens.

Chapter Six
The lactose-free kitchen

If you want complete control over the amount of lactose you eat, you'll find it in your own kitchen.

First, head into your kitchen and carefully examine the items you have in your cupboards, refrigerator and freezer. You may be surprised at how much lactose is lurking in your kitchen. You can remove the items all at once, if you're willing to go all the way, or you can do it in phases. (I recommend doing the job in phases.)

Many of the suggestions in Chapter Five for making food choices when you eat out will also apply to lactose-free home cooking.

Lactose-free home cooking

Cooking lactose free requires a change of thinking. The simpler you cook the better. Use herbs and seasonings to flavor meat, fish, and vegetables. Stick to fresh ingredients and use fewer prepared foods. Experiment with chicken stock or lactose-free milks to make sauces.

Explore cuisines—such as Mediterranean, Indian or Asian—as we discussed; they don't rely very much on dairy products. Once you find a few good recipes, you're well on your way to cooking lactose-free.

Milk

All kinds of milk should be removed, whether low-fat or fortified.

Cheeses

Remove all cheeses for now; there may be some varieties you can add back later.

Yogurts

Toss out all but *unpasteurized* yogurt, or make your own homemade yogurt.

Pancake mixes, cake mixes

These items are sometimes the highest in lactose. Check the labels.

Ice cream

Ice cream isn't a healthy choice because it contains a lot of fat in addition to the lactose. Manufacturers often add even more lactose to make it creamier. So while you're eliminating ice cream because of the lactose it contains, you can also take heart in the fact that you're ridding your diet of something that could clog your arteries and contribute to cardiovascular disease.

Butter and margarine products

You can keep substitute products that are not derived from milk, like sunflower butter, or margarine.

Cream of all kinds

Eliminate cream. This includes products like half-and-half, full cream, whipped cream, heavy whipping cream and low-fat cream.

Remember, give yourself some breathing room

Again, make these lifestyle changes in a slow and controlled manner. Now that you know how prevalent lactose is in food products, you'll need to take some time to look for substitutes. Go at your own pace and you'll stay motivated. For example, you could clean out your pantry slowly, finding lactose-free substitutes one at a time. Remember, if you try to do too much too fast, you could end up in burnout.

Think about giving to others

If you don't want to throw away food, share your items with friends and family or, better yet, give your nonperishable items to a food bank. You'll be able to feel better and feel good at the same time.

Learning to Cook with Non-Dairy Ingredients

The idea of cooking without cheese, cream, butter and other dairy ingredients might seem daunting at first. That's why making a drastic and immediate shift is hard. After being so accustomed to cooking with dairy products, it may take a while to move in a lactose-free direction.

I suggest you start with easy–to-make, lactose-free recipes from experienced chefs, and then work your way to converting your own recipes. You'll find delicious, dairy-free recipes for breakfast, lunch dinner and more in Part Two, which will be a great way to ease yourself into lactose-free cooking.

And, learning new dairy-free recipes could be the key that unlocks a significantly different way of cooking for you. It might be the motivation that exposes you and your family to a new world of tastes and textures. In fact, leaving the dairy-filled world of cooking behind might surprise you. There's an entire world of culinary delights waiting for you.

Adapting you own recipes

If you're willing to adjust things a bit, you can cook your own lactose-friendly meals that your family will love. (They may not even realize you've taken out the dairy.) Remember that using dairy products in your cooking is just one way to prepare meals. As mentioned, many people around the world don't use dairy on a regular basis and still prepare sumptuous meals.

Help for making good choices

You may face some challenges cooking all-out lactose free. Here are some techniques for overcoming these stumbling blocks:

Use milk substitutes in your recipes

One trick is to take advantage of the many milk substitutes that are available. Next time you visit the grocery store, head over to the section that has alternative milk selections.

As mentioned in Chapter Four, you'll quickly see that you have many options for non-dairy milk. There are so many choices, in fact, you might feel a bit overwhelmed by the sheer number. You'll find soy, almond, rice, and coconut milk in the grocery section. Check out health food stores for less well-known choices like oat, cashew nut and hemp milk.

In addition to good taste, you'll also have the flexibility to decide what items work for you in any given dish or recipe. Giving up cow's milk is a lot more palatable with so many alternatives. You might like to use almond milk as an ingredient in a cake, or soy milk in fruit smoothies.

Note: It may take some time for you to re-engineer your own favorite recipes. But, through trial and error, you'll find what works for you and your family.

Go for lean meats and vegetables

When preparing meals, all you really need for a healthy diet are lean meats, vegetables and dairy-free substitutes. Going lactose-free doesn't mean you have to give up chicken, fish and pork for example.

Look for kosher food products at the grocery store

As mentioned in Chapter Five, kosher food is based on the laws of the Jewish religion. Besides other dietary restrictions, Jewish law forbids the mixing of meat and milk at a meal. No dairy by-products of any kind are allowed in kosher meat products sold at grocery stores. Look for the kosher symbol. Most pre-packaged kosher foods have some kind of kosher certification.

Hebrew National is a well-known brand you may have seen that sells only kosher products. They specialize in hotdogs, deli meats and knockwurst. While I'm not saying that hotdogs, for example, offer the best nutrition, if you want a hotdog, consider a kosher one and go lactose free.

Spice things up

Try different calorie-free flavorings and different spices to change things up. You might be surprised by how much you can improve the taste of a dish by giving up dairy products and, instead, adding other ingredients.

When it's all about the cheese

Probably one of the biggest stumbling blocks for many cooks is learning how to cook without cheese. Many recipes revolve around cheese, so this may be the toughest challenge when going lactose free. Fortunately, the growing number of vegans in this country has convinced manufactures to make more alternative products.

Vegans eat nothing sourced from animals. That means no milk, no eggs and definitely no cheese and dairy products. Most vegans eat alternative cheeses. Manufacturers call this kind of cheese "vegan cheese" and it's made mostly from oils like palm oil. Soy and other nondairy cheese alternatives are also available.

The best and most effective way to use vegan cheese is to add chunks or grated portions of it to a hot dish. When you add vegan cheese to a hot dish, the heat breaks down the cheese and improves the appearance of it to make it more appetizing. I don't think it tastes nearly has good as the real thing, but it can be an acceptable option. Give it a try.

One example—pasta the alternative way

Since all the usual tricks of your trade—like butter, cream and cheese—are now out of the question, and many commercial pasta sauces already have cheese in them, you'll need to make your pasta sauce from scratch.

Before, this would have been a doable and, perhaps, enjoyable task. But now that you're cooking lactose-free, the issue is a bit more muddled. All the usual ingredients are no longer available to you. What can you do?

Research

I did a simple search on Google using the keywords "nondairy pasta recipes." Many tasty-sounding recipes came up including Pasta with Parsley-Walnut Pesto, Easy Lasagna and "Creamy" Basil Pasta.

If you want to experiment yourself, you might find other good ideas for making the pasta more appealing using ingredients you like. You can look for cheese alternatives that appeal to you, and consider other topping choices you might have (like freshly cut tomatoes, olives, crushed nuts, red peppers, olive oil, and sun dried tomatoes).

What kind of nuts should you add to pasta? That's entirely up to you. Most common nuts are great for pasta; you can mix and match. I particularly like pine nuts. I brown them lightly in a pan before adding them to a recipe.

Do you want some oil in your pasta? Skip the butter and use extra virgin olive oil instead. If you add two to three tablespoons of oil to your pasta, you'll see that it comes alive with moisture and flavor. Pine nuts go particularly well with olive oil. The best part about making pasta this way? It's great for your heart and other organs because olive oil doesn't add to your levels of bad cholesterol, and it provides energy to you as well.

With these concessions and changes, preparing pasta will be easy again. And the best part—once you've changed the recipe to a lactose-free one, you'll never have to experiment with it again unless you want to.

Keep in mind that lactose-free cooking isn't about restrictions, but about relevant substitutions that add more great ideas and recipes to your kitchen. Don't focus on what you can't eat or cook, but focus on what you can add to your meals. There are an unlimited number of gastronomic delights waiting for you outside the dairy-filled traditional way of cooking.

The more you know, and the more you learn, the more quickly you can make the adjustment to cooking lactose free. Soon the new information will gel, and you'll automatically be making good choices.

Not feeling motivated?

If you find that you're losing motivation, think about your health. Dairy products have needed calcium, to be sure, but most dairy products are also loaded with fat and salt. Most of us already get too much cholesterol, fat and salt in our diets.

If you think about it this way, you can see how there's no need to add more of these unhealthy food items to your diet and how it might be nice to cut them out instead.

We'll talk more about the benefits of calcium and where to find it in a lactose-free world in Chapter Seven.

A family affair

It makes sense for you to cook with non-dairy ingredients in order to avoid lactose, but if you're the only person in your family who's lactose intolerant, you might get some pretty vocal feedback when you first begin cooking lactose-free meals. Children and adults alike love butter, milk and cheese.

The reality is this: You can't force people to eat what you eat, even if the "other people" are your children or your spouse. What can you do then? First, understand your kids' and your spouse's perspective. The reason they may be protesting is because they don't have the need, as you do, for a lactose-free lifestyle. You're suffering from painful and unwelcome symptoms and need to make these drastic changes, but it's not the same for them. Certainly the age of your children will come into play. Teenagers might give you the most push-back.

Educate the family

Explain to your family what lactose intolerance is and what happens to you when you consume products that contain lactose. You may want to use this book to help you explain why you can't ingest the lactose in the foods you eat.

Let your children and spouse know that your condition is likely permanent. Because lactase production decreases over time, the idea that you'll suddenly produce more lactase is unlikely.

It's important that your family members understand that you aren't trying to get them interested in a newfangled diet; you're going to eat lactose-free because you need to be well, and you can't be well if you keep eating dairy products. After giving your family a thorough explanation about your medical condition, it's time to ask them for their input. You can ask what they think about your ailment and how they can help you to eat lactose-free food.

It's important that you emphasize your need for your family's help and that you know they're up to the challenge. You may be surprised to discover how helpful your children can be when they're asked to help Mom or Dad. Once they understand that this is not about them—you want them to enjoy what they eat—it's about you, the amount of cooperation you see may be astonishing.

Once your children understand that you want and need their help, it's time to talk about meals. Ask the following questions; your family's answers might help you gauge how in tune they are with lactose-free foods:

- Would you like to try pasta toppings like pine nuts instead of cheese?

- Are you willing to try soy milk or other kinds of milk alternatives?

- How does the idea of cooking with olive oil instead of butter sound to you?

You can slowly draw your family into the idea of eating food that's lactose free. They probably won't like everything you offer but, as they become more accustomed to eating lactose free, they may welcome new dishes and even ask for more.

Everyone's tastes are different. Some people like adding vinegar and olive oil to salads (lactose free) while others enjoy adding big chunks of cheese. This is a case where your family can have the cheese version if they like, and you can stick to the olive oil and vinegar options.

There might be days when you have to cook a few more items to satisfy your family's craving for dairy. When this happens, you can enjoy your lactose-free food while your family gets their dairy fix.

Most of us aren't keen on the idea of doing double work in the kitchen, particularly if the extra work means cooking both lactose-free and dairy dishes. Compromise is a great solution.

One idea—keep a calendar

Use a calendar to schedule meals throughout the week. You may want to post it on the refrigerator. For example, you can make Monday pasta night and you can tell your family you're going to make the pasta with garlic and nut topping, or olive oil, basil and fresh tomatoes or black olives, or other nondairy items that may appeal to them. Of course they can always sprinkle cheese on top of the pasta.

They might groan a bit, but then they can see that you're making macaroni and cheese on Tuesday. This kind of compromise can keep your family happy. On Tuesday, when the family is enjoying macaroni and cheese, you can enjoy a salad with all of your favorite toppings, or even leftovers from the night before.

Remember that meat is still on the menu for you. Unless you're a vegetarian or vegan, you can enjoy all manner of meats and other proteins.

Chapter Seven
Got Vitamin D, Calcium and the B Vitamins?

Many people think that calcium and vitamin D—the two nutrients most associated with strong teeth and normal bone growth—can only be found in milk. But, thankfully, that's not the case. And there are other sources for the vital B vitamins found in milk as well.

Once you've made the commitment to go completely lactose free, it's *essential* to make sure you get these same nutrients from other sources. Fortunately, there's a simple way to keep track of the amounts of nutrients you need and what you consume every day.

The difference between fat-soluble vitamins and water-soluble ones

Fat-soluble vitamins—namely vitamins A, D, E and K—dissolve in fat and are stored in fat throughout the body. It's difficult for your body to excrete excess fat-soluble vitamins, so toxic levels can accumulate if you consume too many.

Water-soluble vitamins are those that dissolve in water upon entering the body. Because of this, your body can't store excess amounts of water-soluble vitamins for later use. There are a total of nine water-soluble vitamins: the B vitamins—folate, thiamine, riboflavin, niacin, pantothenic acid, biotin, vitamin B6 and vitamin B12—and vitamin C.

Know the IU or the mg

The International Unit (IU) is the global standard for measuring fat-soluble vitamins. It reflects the potency of each vitamin based on the quantity.

Water-soluble vitamins (and minerals like calcium) are measured in milligrams (mg) and micrograms (mcg). One milligram (1/1000 of a gram) is equal to 1000 micrograms.

Know the RDA

RDA stands for the recommended daily allowance of all nutrients and vitamins. These recommendations can vary based on things such as a person's age, gender, illness, past surgeries, the need for dialysis, or other factors. You should know your personal RDA for each of the vitamins, minerals and nutrients your body requires. The RDA values listed here are for the average man and woman.

Getting vitamins and minerals from foods sources first

The B vitamins

Unfortunately, when you give up milk, you're also giving up an easy way to get B vitamins, which are crucial for your body to function properly.

Vitamin B complex is a group of eight vitamins that are critical nutrients for all things mind-related. Mood, memory—even migraines—can benefit from the B's. In the right amounts, the B's can quell anxiety, lift depression, ease PMS and boost your energy.

These B vitamins are a chemically related family of nutrients that work as a team. Their mood-boosting and other health benefits result from intricate behind-the-scenes work in the body.

Some B vitamins help cells burn fats and glucose for energy. Others help make neurotransmitters like serotonin. And some B's assist with the production and repair of DNA.

Many of us don't get enough B's according to the USDA (United States Department of Agriculture). Deficiencies in folic acid, B12, and B6 are especially common.

For information about your country, consult the European Food Safety Authority (EFSA) or other appropriate websites.

Ensuring that your diet contains plenty of nondairy B-rich foods is critical. But if your stress level is high or your mood feels off-kilter, or if your diet is low in B's, you can benefit from the higher amounts present in vitamin B supplements. (See Chapter Eight.)

One American research group found that, over the course of a two-year study, large doses of vitamins B6, B12 and folic acid reduced shrinkage of the brain by thirty percent.

Food Sources:

Vitamin B6

Poultry, fish and organ meats are all rich in vitamin B6. Other major sources of vitamin B6 are potatoes and other starchy vegetables. Fruit (other than citrus) is also among the major sources of vitamin B6.

The recommended daily allowance for B6 for adults from nineteen to fifty years old is 1.3 mg (milligrams). For people over fifty, the RDA is 1.7 mg for men, and 1.5 mg for women.

Vitamin B12

Vitamin B12 can be found in beef liver and clams, which are the best sources of this essential vitamin. Fish, meat, poultry and eggs also contain vitamin B12. Many breakfast cereals are also fortified with vitamin B12. Check the labels.

The recommended RDA for B12 is 2.4 mcg (micrograms) for both men and women fourteen or older.

Folic acid

Folic acid is the synthetic form of folate. You can find folate in a wide variety of foods including vegetables (especially dark green leafy vegetables like spinach and turnip greens), fruits and fruit juices, nuts, beans, peas, poultry, meat, eggs, seafood and grains. Spinach, liver, yeast, asparagus and Brussels sprouts are among the foods with the highest levels of folate.

In 1996, the United States FDA (Food and Drug Administration) published regulations requiring the addition of folic acid to enriched breads, cereals, flours, corn meals, pastas, rice, and other grain products. Since cereals and grains are widely consumed in the U.S., these products have become a very important contributor of folic acid to the American diet. However, check these products for lactose before you purchase any of them.

Outside the U.S., check with the European Food Safety Authority (EFSA) or other appropriate agency.

The recommended RDA for folic acid is 400 mcg for both men and women fourteen and older.

Calcium

Calcium is the most common mineral in the human body. About ninety-nine percent of the calcium in the body is found in bones and teeth, while the other one percent is present in the blood and soft tissue.

Calcium is an essential nutrient. It's a crucial component in maintaining strong and healthy teeth and bones. It's also required, at the molecular level, in many biological processes in the body.

The body needs calcium for muscles to move and for nerves to carry messages between the brain and every body part. Proper amounts of calcium help keep your joints free of inflammation and arthritis as well as help your muscles contract.

Calcium also keeps your blood pressure normal, and reduces the risk of colon cancer. In addition, calcium is used to help blood vessels move blood throughout the body and to help release hormones and enzymes that affect almost every function in the human body.

Your body stores excess calcium until you reach your early thirties—the time you reach your peak bone density. After that, your body stops storing calcium and you must rely on getting all the calcium you need from your diet. If you don't, you'll deplete the calcium stores in your body. It's like taking all the money out of a piggy bank and not putting any back in. You end up penniless.

As your body depletes the calcium stored in your bones, they become weaker and weaker until finally they're almost hollow. These fragile bones are much easier to break.

Some depressing news

Because of their calcium-depleted bones, many older women suffer hip fractures, which can be extremely debilitating. Case in point, many of the 300,000 hip fractures that occur each year in the United States happen in postmenopausal women with fragile bones.

Researchers have found that women age sixty-five and older, who fracture a hip, are much more likely to die during the following year than they would be if they had avoided injury.

The increased risk of death associated with hip fractures, researchers found, was especially dramatic among women in the sixty-five- to sixty-nine-year-old age group; the odds of death were five times higher for women after a fracture than they were for non-injured women of the same age.

Thinning of the bones is silent. It doesn't hurt, and if you're not proactive you might not know you have it until you break something. Your doctor can order a bone density test. (See more information about the bone density test in Chapter Eight.)

To keep our bones young, men need 1,000 to 1,200 milligrams of calcium each day; women under sixty need about 1,200 milligrams. Women over the age of sixty need 1,600 milligrams of calcium a day to keep their bones the youngest and strongest possible.

How to get calcium if you're lactose intolerant

Of course, the easiest sources of calcium are milk and other dairy products. When your restrict dairy in your diet, you're also restricting calcium. So if you need to completely abandon milk and other dairy products because of your lactose intolerance, the question becomes how can you get the calcium you need?

To start with—go green

Some plant sources provide great ways to get calcium. Vegetables like kale, cabbages, broccoli, and collard greens are a great source of calcium.

You'll find a number of other natural sources of calcium you can try as you progressively adapt to your new lactose-free lifestyle. You might not like everything on this list, but you'll probably find a few vegetables or some other food items that will give you enough calcium and, at the same time, will satisfy your appetite and taste.

Source	Amount of calcium
Artichoke (medium-sized)	25 milligrams
8 ounces lentils	38 milligrams
Almond butter (1 tbsp.)	43 milligrams
Tortilla (6-inch)	45 milligrams
Wheat bread (2 slices)	60 milligrams
Orange (medium-sized)	61 milligrams
8 ounces broccoli	62 milligrams
8 ounces garbanzos	77 milligrams
Blackstrap molasses (1 tbsp.)	82 milligrams
8 ounces kidney beans	87 milligrams
8 ounces kale	95 milligrams
1 ounce sour cream (nondairy)	100 milligrams
8 ounces pinto beans	103 milligrams
8 ounces mustard greens	104 milligrams

4 ounces dried figs	121 milligrams
Tahini (2 tbsp.)	128 milligrams
8 ounces bok choy	158 milligrams
8 ounces soy cheese	183 milligrams
84 grams salmon	188 milligrams
8 ounces almond milk (fortified)	200 milligrams
28 grams soy cheese (fortified)	300 milligrams
8 ounces turnip greens	209 milligrams
8 ounces collard greens	266 milligrams
16 ounces yogurt (soy-based)	299 milligrams
8 ounces fortified orange juice	300 milligrams
8 ounces fortified rice milk	300 milligrams
8 ounces fortified soy milk	300 milligrams
4 ounces tofu	434 milligrams

Go for the grains

Most grains don't have high amounts of calcium unless they're fortified. But because most people eat them on a regular basis, their calcium contribution can add up.

The good news is that once you find good, natural sources of calcium, your body will be able to absorb calcium more easily than from cow's milk.

Vitamin D

Roughly half of adults — older adults in particular — don't get enough vitamin D. What are the implications? This micronutrient is essential to our muscles, bones and immune system. If you don't get enough vitamin D, you may be at risk for vitamin D deficiency. It's a real concern because new research links low levels of vitamin D to a growing list of health problems, including heart disease and cancer.

Decreased or insufficient levels of vitamin D have been linked to:

- Cancer — Research suggests that vitamin D may help protect against breast, prostate and colon cancer

- Diabetes — Vitamin D may reduce the risk for type I diabetes in children

- Heart disease — Low blood levels of vitamin D may be related to cardiovascular disease

- Osteoporosis — Low levels of vitamin D have been tied to osteoporosis and hip fractures in older women. (We'll talk more about osteoporosis in Chapter Eight.)

- Suppressed immunity: Without adequate vitamin D, we have increased susceptibility to infectious agents.

- Heightened inflammation: Vitamin D is a key cofactor in regulating inflammation throughout the body.

With all of these findings, researchers point out that further investigation is needed, but they project that the incidence of some diseases could be reduced by twenty to fifty percent or more if vitamin D deficiency was eliminated.

Milk has it

Did you know that approximately three and a half cups of whole, reduced-fat or non-fat milk can give you all the Vitamin D your body needs for an entire day? So, the question becomes, "If I can't drink milk, where do I get the Vitamin D I need?"

Easy. We'll talk about food sources in a bit, but let's start with the greatest source of vitamin D of all—the sun. Vitamin D is produced naturally by your body following exposure to sunlight. If you get a healthy dose of sunlight each day, you can synthesize your own vitamin D in an incredibly natural way.

You definitely need D

Did you know the human body actually can't live without vitamin D? For hundreds of thousands of years, our ancestors lived with the sun—spending far more time outdoors than they did indoors. Because of this, we humans developed a dependence on sunshine for health and life, including the ability to get essential vitamin D from the sun.

Because sunlight *alone* can bring your vitamin D levels into the healthy range, it's important to get the right amount of sun exposure to help your body produce this essential vitamin.

Sun exposure the healthy way

Vitamin D is known as the "sunshine vitamin" because the ultraviolet rays from the sunlight strike the skin causing vitamin D to be made. If you expose your arms and legs to the sun for a short period of time (well before you burn) your body will produce between 2,000 and 4,000 IU of vitamin D. In a bathing suit, the dose jumps to between 10,000 and 25,000 IU.

To put this in context, the RDA of vitamin D is based on age. For people one to seventy years old, 600 IU is recommended daily. For those seventy years and older, 800 IU per day is recommended daily. For pregnant and nursing women, 600 IU daily is the recommendation.

You may be thinking, "Wait a minute, if I get vitamin D from the sun, won't I get way over the recommended amount?"

Although it's possible, in rare instances, to take an overdose of a vitamin D *supplement*, you can't overdose on vitamin D when you get it from the sun. Our bodies contain a built-in mechanism which allows us to manufacture exactly the right amount of vitamin D we need from the sun—no more—no less.

We've all heard the warnings about the dangers of sun exposure—from premature aging to skin cancer, and we should take those warnings *extremely* seriously. But, experts say, you can get the sun you need—far less than you may think—and be safe, too. Very little sun exposure is needed to provide your body's needs.

Put yourself out there

To get vitamin D from the sun, make a plan and do what you can. Run or play tennis or volleyball, or go to the beach. Swim, water ski, bike, hike—you get the idea.

If you don't want to commit to that much time and energy, there are lots of other things you can do. Sit on your front porch, go for a walk, roll down the windows when you drive, or even open the windows in your house and find a sunny corner to sit in. You'll most likely find a way to fit in your sun time.

How much is not too much?

Here's a general rule: If there's enough sunlight to cause a reddening of your skin when you're outside for any length of time, then there are enough UVB (ultraviolet) rays to assist your body in making vitamin D.

Estimate the time it would take for your skin to turn pink in the sun. Then divide that time by 25 to 50 percent, depending on your skin type. Obviously someone with fair skin will need to spend less time in the sun than someone with darker skin.

Sunscreen is a must

If you want to stay outdoors longer than the specified time, be sure to wear sunscreen. While it's important not to wear sunscreen during your "Vitamin D—enhancing times" (a sunscreen with an SPF as low as eight can block as much as ninety-five percent of vitamin D production) sunscreen is a MUST at all other times. It's essential to protect your skin. And, if you needed more convincing—if your skin starts to turn red—you're not going to enhance your vitamin D levels anyway.

Did you know that experts recommend keeping sunscreen on your face even if you're indoors? It may seem excessive, but even sunlight filtered through your windows is enough to damage your skin.

Suzanne's sun story

Take a look at a personal story. Suzanne has fair skin, burns easily and lives in Chicago, Illinois, United States. Chicago's coordinates are 41°52'55"N and 87°27'40"W. To put that in context, Italy, Spain, Turkey, Armenia, Albania and Greece are also located at or near this latitude.

Suzanne should spend twenty to thirty minutes in the sun with her arms and legs exposed (but not her face) between the hours of 11 a.m. and 3 p.m. two to three times a week from March through May and September through October, but only fifteen to twenty minutes in July and August when the sun in strongest.

She shouldn't even try to get sun time from November through February in her area; she wouldn't get enough UV to help, and she'd probably get pretty cold outside with bare arms and legs.

Stocking up

If you can maintain a sun schedule for your individual needs, you'll probably get enough UVB (ultraviolet) rays to keep your bone mass intact all year long because your body can stockpile vitamin D for use during low-sunlight times.

Our bodies needed to develop this ability to stockpile vitamin D because, of course, not all regions of the earth are equal when it comes to ultraviolet exposure. (Think Miami versus Michigan or Mexico versus Montreal.)

Remember, the more skin you expose, the quicker you make vitamin D. But, don't get any sun on your face without using sunscreen; it'll cause premature aging and wrinkles.

Older people need more sun exposure

As we age, our bodies become less efficient at making our own vitamin D. So if you're older than sixty-five, you may need more time in the sun to get the same benefit.

How to have your sun and be safe, too

It's all a matter of balance—not too much sun, not too little. Get outdoors on a regular basis. The benefits of even small amounts of UVB (ultraviolet) light are so remarkable that scientists are studying the effects of providing artificial UVB light to seniors. And NASA is looking into installing artificial UVB light into spaceships for long missions to counteract the effects of weightlessness on bone.

Since this is the way Nature intended, make the sun your method of choice.

But what do you do when you can't get enough sunlight?

If you can't get vitamin D from the sun, you must get it from your diet. While it's difficult to get the high levels of vitamin D you need without the sun, you can get enough vitamin D from foods and supplements to help build and maintain bone mass. Remember that sunlight is more reliable than any food or supplement.

Food sources of vitamin D

Good food sources of vitamin D are liver; cod liver oil; egg yolks and oily fish; such as salmon, tuna, and sardines.

There are other ways to get your daily dose of vitamin D. Did you know that many brands of orange juice have been fortified with vitamin D? When you drink these brands, you're not only getting a healthy dose of the very beneficial vitamin C, but also other vitamins and minerals including the necessary vitamin D.

Do read labels, however. You want to make sure that the orange juice you choose has been fortified (vitamin D is not naturally found in orange juice). If you don't buy the fortified brands, you'll only get the nutrients found in regular (non-fortified) concentrates and juices.

You can also look at milk alternatives. The soy milk I drink is also fortified with vitamin D, as are some other nondairy products. It may take a little detective work, but you should be able to put together enough food products along with vitamin D supplements to get the daily dose of vitamin D you need. (For more information on supplements, see Chapter Eight.)

Chapter Eight
Got Supplements?

In addition to eating a diet rich in the necessary nutrients, take a look at supplements as a way to round out your diet.

Essential vitamins, such as the B vitamins (B12, B6 and folic acid) and vitamin D, as mentioned, are available in supplement form. You'll also find minerals like calcium offered as supplements. Often, experts say, supplements can be a better source than dairy to get some of these vital nutrients essential for healthy growth and development.

As a reminder, as we discussed in Chapter Seven, vitamins are separated into two categories—fat soluble and water-soluble—based on how they're absorbed and whether or not they're stored in your body.

Scientific units of measure for supplements

There are different scientific units for measuring the amounts of vitamins and minerals in each soft gel or tablet.

As mentioned in Chapter Seven, an international unit (IU) is the global standard for measuring fat-soluble vitamins (A, D, E and K). Water-soluble vitamins (the B vitamins and minerals like calcium) are measured in milligrams (mg) and micrograms (mcg).

You should know the RDA for every supplement you take. We'll discuss the B vitamins, vitamin D, and calcium supplements later in this chapter. But first, some words of caution.

Supplements may not be what they seem

When you see claims like "miracle cure," "revolutionary scientific breakthrough," or "alternative to drugs or surgery," you should think twice before buying these supplements. These terms should signal a health fraud alert.

Health fraud scams have been around for hundreds of years. The snake oil salesmen of old have morphed into the deceptive, high-tech marketers of today. They prey on people's desires for easy solutions to difficult health problems—from losing weight to curing serious diseases like cancer.

The Food and Drug Administration (FDA) in the United States, and the European Food Safety Authority (EFSA) are charged with protecting consumers from fraudulent claims by manufacturers. (Check for similar agencies in other countries.)

A health product is fraudulent if it is deceptively promoted as being effective against a disease or health condition, but has not been scientifically proven safe and effective for that purpose.

Scammers promote their products through newspapers, magazines, TV infomercials and cyberspace. You can find health fraud scams in retail stores and on countless websites, in popup ads and spam, and on social media sites like Facebook and Twitter.

Not worth the risk

Health fraud scams can do more than waste your money; they can cause serious injury or even death. If you use an unproven treatment, it can delay you getting a potentially life-saving diagnosis and medication that actually works. Also, fraudulent products sometimes contain hidden drug ingredients that can be harmful when unknowingly taken by consumers.

Fraudulent products often make claims related to:

- weight loss

- sexual performance

- memory loss

- serious diseases such as cancer, diabetes, heart disease, arthritis and Alzheimer's

A pervasive problem

In the past few years, for example, FDA laboratories have found more than 100 weight-loss products, illegally marketed as "dietary supplements," that contained sibutramine, the active ingredient in the prescription weight-loss drug Meridia. In 2010, Meridia was withdrawn from the U.S. market after studies showed that it was associated with an increased risk of heart attack and stroke.

Health fraud is a pervasive problem especially when scammers sell online. It's difficult to track down the responsible parties. Some manufacturers will comply when told their products are illegal and will shut down their websites. Unfortunately, however, these same products may reappear later on a different website, and sometimes with a different name.

The FDA and the EFSA post alerts on their websites for new supplements that come on the market that carry risks for the consumer. Before you decide to take a new unconventional supplement, check these websites for any alerts.

B vitamins, vitamin D and calcium

Having said all that, if you do a little research, you should have no difficulty in finding conventional supplements, like the B's, D and calcium, from reputable manufacturers in drug stores, health food stores and some retail outfits. But if you choose to go online, that's when you have to be careful. The point is to do the research and know exactly what you're getting and from whom. Look to manufacturers you trust.

Some vitamin and mineral supplements have the potential to interact with prescription and over-the-counter medications you may be taking. Be sure to check with your doctor or pharmacist before adding any supplement to your diet.

RDA for B's, D and calcium

As noted in Chapter Seven, the recommended daily allowance (RDA) of vitamin D is based on age. For people one to seventy years old, 600 IU is recommended daily. For those seventy years and older, 800 IU per day is recommended daily. For pregnant and nursing women, 600 IU daily is the recommendation.

These recommendations are for the optimal absorption of calcium and the optimal incorporation into the bone.

The B vitamins

The recommended amount of vitamin B12 for adults is 2.4 mcg (micrograms). The recommended amount of vitamin B6 for people under fifty-one is 1.3 mg (milligrams). For people over fifty-one the amount is 1.7 mg for men and 1.5 mg for women. The recommended amount of folic acid for adults nineteen and over is 400 mcg.

Calcium Supplements

For bone health, men need 1,000 to 1,200 milligrams of calcium each day; women under sixty need about 1,200 milligrams. Women over the age of sixty need 1,600 milligrams of calcium a day to keep their bones the youngest and strongest possible. (These amounts refer to actual calcium, not calcium combined with citrate or carbonate; if you choose supplements with citrate or carbonate, check the label for the supplement's actual amount of calcium.)

Tip: To make sure calcium is properly absorbed, add an additional 20 milligrams of calcium for every twelve-ounce caffeinated soft drink or four-ounce cup of coffee you drink.

Read labels; choose wisely. You'll want a supplement with 600 milligrams of calcium at a time, plus 200 milligrams of magnesium and 200 IU of vitamin D in a size and taste you can swallow. It may take three or four pills to get the dosage right—whatever works for you. There's more than one way to do it. Just avoid supplements that have iron in them. (Iron inhibits calcium absorption.)

Also, calcium needs an acidic environment for absorption, so if you're getting your calcium in an antacid that neutralizes acid, you're probably not getting an optimal amount.

Why do you need to take 200 IU of vitamin D along with the 200 milligrams of magnesium at the same time you take a calcium supplement? Vitamin D increases the absorption of calcium, making it more efficient in delivering calcium to your bones. Magnesium is also necessary to assist calcium absorption.

So, in general, that means if you take your calcium with 200 IU of vitamin D, you'll still need to add enough additional vitamin D to get the total amount your body needs (600 IU to 800 IU vitamin D) every day.

Calcium gives—but, salt takes away

People in the United States generally need more calcium to maintain strong bones than people in some other countries. The culprit is sitting on the kitchen shelf and it's called salt, or "sodium chloride."

Salt, while tasty, is bad for the human body. We only need about **130 milligrams** of salt each day for normal metabolic functioning, but most of us get much more. A regular bag of potato chips has about **2,200 milligrams** of salt. That's an incredible amount to consume in a short period of time. And your body's capacity to get rid of the excess salt is limited. This excessive salt in the body leaches calcium from the bones.

To rid your body of excess salt, you'll need to drink water by the liter to dilute the salt and flush it from your body. Don't stop drinking as soon as you've quenched your thirst.   It takes a lot more water than that to effectively eliminate the salt.

While potato chips are a common source, salt is present everywhere. So be aware—high quantities of sodium can be found in tomato salsas, biscuits, crackers, cookies, and cheeses.

Other ways to strengthen your bones

Exercise is critical in keeping your bones strong. Lifting weights and doing other resistance training is a perfect way to strengthen your bones. Exercise communicates to the body that it must keep the bones strong; the bones respond by holding on to calcium. You reduce your chance of losing bone density and you ultimately end up with stronger bones if you exercise.

What exactly is resistance training?

You don't need to belong to a gym or have a set of weights to do resistance exercises. Any exercise that causes the muscles to contract against an external resistance will do. The external resistance can be dumbbells, rubber exercise tubing, your own body weight (think pull-ups and pushups), bricks, bottles of water, or any other object that causes the muscles to contract.

You should do some form of resistance exercise at least four times a week for at least forty minutes each time in order to get the full bone-building benefits.

Tip: Remember that bones need vitamin D, as well as calcium to stay strong and resist fractures. As previously mentioned in Chapter Seven, you can get enough vitamin D by getting the proper amount of sunlight each day. So, if you exercise outdoors, you can get a combination of vitamin D and bone-building benefits. It's two for one.

Again, you can find extensive information on supplements at the U.S National Institutes of Health—Office of Dietary Supplements website, the FDA's website and the EFSA in Europe.

Osteoporosis

Without sufficient vitamin D and calcium, you're at risk for osteoporosis. The word "osteoporosis" literally means "porous bones." It occurs when bones lose an excessive amount of their protein and mineral content, particularly calcium. Over time, bone mass and bone strength decreases. As a result, bones become fragile and break easily. Even a sneeze or a sudden movement may be enough to break a bone in someone with severe osteoporosis. Although the condition is often considered a "women's disease," men also are affected to a lesser degree.

By the way, I confirmed the definition of osteoporosis at a medical dictionary website. Right next to the definition was an ad for a "proven natural wonder drug" to cure osteoporosis. Remember "caveat emptor" or buyer beware.

Bone density test

Many people don't know they have osteoporosis until they have a fracture or have a bone density scan, also known as a bone mineral density (BMD) test. A bone density scan is a simple, non-invasive test that measures your bone density or volume of calcium and minerals within bone tissue. Bone density scans can help to:

- Detect osteoporosis before you have a fracture

- Predict your chance of fracturing in the future

- Determine your rate of bone loss or monitor the effects of treatment

A bone density scan requires little preparation. You can eat normally and take medications as prescribed by your doctor the morning of your test.

The only restrictions are:

- Don't take any vitamin pills or mineral supplements the morning of your exam.

- You must not have had any exams involving barium or radioisotopes within the last month. These scans interfere with the bone density results.

How it works

The bone density test measures bone loss by exposing parts of the body to ionizing radiation, which electrically charges atoms and molecules. When the exam is being performed in a clinic or radiology room, you'll lie on a padded table that is lit from below, similar to a tanning booth. A medical imager passes over the body without touching it. The large lit arm sends radiation through the body, equal to about one-tenth of the amount of radiation received in a typical chest X-ray.

The entire procedure takes about 10 minutes. A smaller portable device can be used on the hand or foot to measure bone density. Portable bone scans often are provided by pharmacies and, though helpful, they're not as accurate as full-body or hip and leg bone scans.

A last word on supplements

Know your recommended daily allowance for each supplement and read the labels. Because high doses of some supplements can have risks, how do you know when it's okay to take more than the RDA?

One way is to look for the UL (tolerable upper intake level) of a nutrient. In the U.S., the Institute of Medicine sets the UL after reviewing studies of that nutrient.

With many vitamins and minerals, you can safely take a dose much higher than the RDA without coming close to the UL. For instance, the average person can take more than 50 times the RDA of vitamin B6 without reaching the upper limit. However, some people develop neuropathy symptoms (damage to certain nerves) with these higher levels of B6. So you should always be cautious. Here are some things to keep in mind:

Some supplements are riskier than others. With some vitamins and minerals, the upper limit is pretty close to the RDA. So it's easy to get too much. For example, a man taking just over three times the RDA of vitamin A would be taking more than the upper limit. High doses of vitamin A—and other fat-soluble vitamins like E and K—can build up in the body and cause toxicity. Other risky supplements include the minerals iron and selenium.

The UL is often the limit for *all* sources of a nutrient. It can include the amount you get from *both food and supplements*. So when figuring out whether you're reaching the UL on a particular nutrient, you usually need to factor in the food you eat. You won't find the UL on food nutrition labels or on your vitamin bottle. It's not a number that most people know about. But it's available on the appropriate government websites.

To be on the safe side, stay below the UL for any nutrient. And if you have a health condition, check with your health care provider before taking supplements. As mentioned, some supplements can have possible drug interactions and side effects.

The good news is that the average person is unlikely to take so much of a nutrient that he or she will run into trouble. But it's always wise to check in with a doctor before you start using a supplement regularly. And that's definitely true if you're using any supplement in high doses or for prolonged periods of time.

Your magnificent body

Finally, remember that the human body is an amazing creation and it can adapt to changes. The human body ultimately knows how to take care of itself—we just need to support it as we let it do its job. Let your body acclimate to your needs and you'll be amazed by how well it can and will adapt to your changing lifestyle and new eating habits.

In Part Two, you'll discover some incredibly mouthwatering recipes you can enjoy as you live lactose free. You'll find that living the lactose-free lifestyle is not only doable and delicious, it can offer a whole new way of living life to the fullest.

Part Two
Recipes

Lactose-Free Delights

As you know, being lactose intolerant doesn't mean you can't enjoy your favorite foods; you just need to prepare them with lactose-free ingredients.

You'll find some delicious lactose-free recipes here. Enjoy the recipes—improve on them if you'd like—and start making your own meals at home. As you adapt your cooking style, you'll discover freedom from your symptoms and the joy of improving health.

Did you know that there are hundreds of lactose-free recipes available on the internet? The possibilities are endless. Here are just a few.

Bon appetite!

Breakfast

Easy Granola

http://www.drgourmet.com/recipes/breakfast/easyg
ranola.shtml

Servings=6 | Serving size=about 1 cup

Cooking Time = 75 Minutes

This recipe can be multiplied by 2, 3.

Store tightly covered at room temperature. Keeps well for 4-5 days.

Ingredients:

- 3 quarts water
- 1 1/3 cups steel cut oats
- 2/3 cup quinoa
- ¼ cup sliced almonds
- ¼ cup chopped walnuts
- ½ cup unsweetened applesauce

- ½ tsp ground cinnamon

- ½ tsp ground nutmeg

- 1/8 teaspoon salt

- 2 Tbsp pure maple syrup

- ¼ cup raisins

- ¼ cup dried cranberries

Directions

1. Preheat oven to 300°F.

2. Place the water in a large sauce pan over high heat. When the water is boiling add the oats and quinoa. Reduce the heat to a simmer and cook for 12 minutes.

3. Drain and rinse with cold water.

4. Place the drained oats and quinoa in a large bowl with the almonds, walnuts, applesauce, cinnamon, nutmeg, salt, maple syrup, raisins and cranberries.

5. Fold together until well blended.

6. Place on a large cookie sheet lined with aluminum foil. Spread as flat as possible and place in the oven.

7. Bake for 45 minutes. Stir with a fork every 10 to 12 minutes.

8. Remove and let cool fully before storing.

Pumpkin Bread

http://www.rachaelray.com/recipe.php?recipe_id=45
56

Serves 6

Ingredients:

- 1 cup pumpkin, canned, *or* steamed and 1 1/2 cups all-purpose flour

- 1 cup sugar

- 1/2 teaspoon cinnamon

- 1/2 teaspoon cloves

- 1/2 teaspoon nutmeg

- 1/2 teaspoon baking soda

- 1/2 teaspoon baking powder

- 1/4 teaspoon salt

- 1/2 cup unrefined coconut oil, at room temperature

- 1 large egg, whisked, pureed

- 1 cup chopped walnuts

Directions:

1. Pre-heat the oven to 350°F.

2. Grease a loaf pan and coat it with flour.

3. Line the bottom with a piece of parchment paper.

4. In a large bowl, whisk together the flour, sugar, cinnamon, cloves, nutmeg, baking soda, baking powder and salt.

5. In another large bowl, whisk together the oil, egg and pumpkin.

6. Stir the dry ingredients into the pumpkin mixture in two batches.

7. Fold in the walnuts.

8. Bake for 70 minutes, or until a toothpick inserted in the top comes out clean.

9. Cool for 20 minutes, then turn onto a rack and cool completely.

Holiday Brunch Gus-tinis

http://www.rachaelray.com/recipe.php?recipe_id=23 88

Ingredients

- 2 teaspoons extra virgin olive oil (EVOO)

- 2 cloves garlic, finely chopped (for people portions only)

- 5 ounces frozen chopped spinach (half of a 10 ounce box), thawed and squeezed dry

- 1 large egg

- A pinch of ground nutmeg

- 1-2 slices wheat bread, toasted and cut into triangles

- Salt and pepper (for people portions only)

Directions

1. In a medium size nonstick skillet, heat the EVOO over medium heat.

2. Add the garlic and cook until fragrant, 30 seconds.

3. Add the spinach and cook until heated through.

4. Add the egg and stir to scramble, 1-2 minutes.

5. Remove from the heat and stir in the nutmeg.

6. Top the toast with the spinach-egg mixture.

7. Season with salt and pepper.

Bacon Garlic Hash Browns

http://www.drgourmet.com/recipes/breakfast/baconhashbrowns.shtml

Servings = 2 | Serving size =about 1 cup

Cooking Time = 30 Minutes

This recipe can be multiplied by 2, 3, 4, 5, 6, 7, 8

Leftovers are fair – reheat gently.

Ingredients

- 1 strip bacon

- 4 cloves garlic (minced)

- 1 large rib of celery (diced)

- 8 ounces red potatoes (large dice)

- 1/8 tsp salt

- 1 tsp dried sage

- Fresh ground black pepper to (taste)

Directions

1. Place the bacon in a medium skillet over medium-high heat. Cover and cook for 5 minutes, then turn the bacon and continue cooking for another 5 minutes. Reduce the heat if the bacon is browning too quickly.

2. Remove the cooked bacon to a paper towel on a plate. When the bacon cools, mince the bacon and set aside.

3. Add the garlic to the rendered bacon fat in the skillet and sauté 3 minutes, or until soft.

4. Add the celery and continue to cook, stirring frequently, for 3-5 minutes or until the celery is soft.

5. Add the diced potatoes and continue cooking, covered, stirring every 2 minutes, until the potatoes are slightly tender.

6. Add the bacon, sage, salt and pepper, stir, and cook, covered, about 10 minutes or until the potatoes are soft and lightly browned. Serve.

Healthy Fresh Cranberry-Orange-Coconut Muffins

http://www.food.com/recipe/healthy-fresh-cranberry-orange-coconut-muffins-489471

Yields: 16 muffins

Ingredients:

- 1 cup fresh cranberries, chopped

- 1/4 cup sugar

- 1/4 cup brown sugar

- 1/4 cup unsweetened flaked coconut

- 1 1/2 cups white whole wheat flour

- 1/4 cup coconut flour

- 1/4 cup oat bran

- 3 teaspoons baking powder

- 1/2 teaspoon kosher salt

- 1/3 cup coconut butter, melted

- 3/4 cup orange juice

- 2 large eggs

- 1/2 cup pepitas (raw hulled pumpkin seeds)

- Turbinado sugar, for sprinkling on top before baking

Directions:

NOTE: If you're **not** using coconut flour, you can probably use ½ cup instead of ¾ cup of orange juice. Coconut flour requires more liquid.

1. Preheat oven to 400 degrees F.

2. Line muffin tins with paper cups. (The new parchment ones are best.) In a bowl, stir together cranberries and regular sugar.

3. In a large bowl sift together flours, oat bran, coconut flakes, baking powder, salt and brown sugar.

4. Whisk eggs, OJ, and melted butter and then add to dry ingredients all at once and stir until moistened.

5. Fold in sugared cranberries.

6. Scoop into prepared muffins liners evenly.

7. Sprinkle desired amount of Turbinado sugar on top of each.

8. Bake at 400F for 20 minutes or until lightly brown and toothpick comes out cleanly.

Dairy-Free Banana Muffins

http://dairyfreecooking.about.com/od/muffinsbiscuits/r/DairyFree_Banana_Muffins_Recipe.htm

Feel free to add chopped nuts, dark dairy-free chocolate, or anything that suits your palate!

Prep Time: 10 minutes

Cook Time: 25 minutes

Total Time: 35 minutes

Yield: 12 large muffins

Ingredients:

- 1 1/2 cups all-purpose flour

- 3/4 cup white granulated sugar

- 1 t. baking powder

- 1 t. baking soda

- 1/2 t. salt

- 1 1/2 cup mashed bananas (from about 3 large overripe bananas)

- 1 egg

- 1/3 cup canola oil

- 1/4 cup plain soy milk

- 1 t. lemon juice

Directions

1. Preheat the oven to 350 F.

2. Lightly oil a 12-cup muffin tin or line with paper liners.

3. In a large mixing bowl, combine the flour, sugar, baking powder, baking soda and salt. Set aside.

4. In another mixing bowl, combine the mashed bananas, egg, canola oil, soy milk and lemon juice until well mixed.

5. Add the wet ingredients to the dry, mixing until just combined.

6. Bake for 25 to 30 minutes, or until a toothpick inserted into the center of a muffin emerges clean.

7. Allow muffins to cool in the pan for about 15 minutes before transferring to a wire cooling rack to cool completely. Serve warm or at room temperature.

Zucchini Cranberry Muffins

http://www.rachaelray.com/recipe.php?recipe_id=42
28

Makes 10 muffins

Ingredients

- 1 3/4 cups flour

- 1/2 teaspoon baking powder

- 1/2 teaspoon baking soda

- 1/2 teaspoon cinnamon

- 1/2 teaspoon salt

- 2 eggs

- 1/2 cup vegetable oil

- 1 cup sugar

- 1/2 teaspoon vanilla

- 1/2 cup fresh or frozen whole cranberries

- 1 large zucchini

Finely grate to yield 1 cup grated zucchini – be sure to use the small grate holes on the box grater, and soak up excess moisture from grated zucchini with some paper towels.

Directions

1. Pre-heat the oven to 375°F. Spray 10 cups of a muffin pan with nonstick cooking spray.

   In a medium size bowl, whisk together the flour, baking powder, baking soda, cinnamon and salt.

2. In a large bowl, whisk together the eggs, sugar, oil and vanilla. Stir in the zucchini.

3. Add the flour mixture and stir to combine; do not over mix.

4. Using a rubber spatula, fold in the cranberries.

5. Divide the batter evenly among the prepared muffin cups.

6. Bake, rotating the pan halfway through, until a toothpick inserted in a muffin comes out clean, 24-28 minutes.

7. Let cool in the pan for 10 minutes, and then turn out the muffins to cool completely.

Pumpkin Oatmeal

http://low-cholesterol.food.com/recipe/pumpkin-oatmeal-102176

Yields: One serving

Ingredients:

1. 1/2 cup old fashioned oats (example Quaker oats)

2. 1 cup water

3. 1/8 cup pumpkin

4. 1 teaspoon pumpkin pie spice

5. 1 tablespoon brown sugar

6. 1 (1 g) packet Splendid sugar substitute

Directions:

1. In a bowl, combine all ingredients.

2. Add some chopped nuts, if desired.

3. Microwave oatmeal for 2-3 minutes depending on your microwave

4. Be careful of the oatmeal boiling over.

5. This could also be done on a stovetop, campfire, or in a slow cooker. Give your oatmeal a good stir.

French Toast (gluten-free, lactose & casein-free)

http://www.food.com/recipe/french-toast-gluten-free-lactose-casein-free-203497

Yields: 2 Servings

Ingredients:

- 2 medium eggs

- 2 tablespoons orange juice

- ¼ cup almond milk (plain or vanilla) or ¼ cup rice milk (plain or vanilla) or ¼ cup soymilk (plain or vanilla)

- ¼ teaspoon cinnamon

- 1/8 teaspoon nutmeg

- ¼ teaspoon salt

- ¼ teaspoon vanilla extract

- 2 tablespoons ghee or 2 tablespoons margarine

- 4 slices gluten-free bread

Optional

2 teaspoons honey

Directions:

1. Whisk together all ingredients except ghee/butter/margarine and bread in a pie pan or small baking dish until thoroughly blended.

2. Heat ghee, butter or margarine in non-stick pan or griddle over medium-high heat.

3. If you're using a dense bread, such as those from "Food for Life," Soak for 3-5 minutes on each side.

4. If you're using homemade bread or a softer or more crumbly bread, soak for only 1-2 minutes on each side.

5. Using a fork or tongs, remove each slice of bread from the liquid and allow excess liquid to drip off.

6. Place in hot ghee/butter/margarine and cook on each side until browned.

7. Serve immediately with maple syrup, jam and/or fresh fruit.

Gluten-and lactose-free bread

http://www.food.com/recipe/gluten-lactose-free-bread-57170

Yields: One loaf

Dry Ingredients:

- 2 cups rice flour
- 1/2 cup potato starch
- 1/2 cup tapioca flour
- 1/3 cup cornstarch
- 1 tablespoon xanthan gum
- 1 1/2 teaspoons salt
- 3 tablespoons granulated sugar
- 1 tablespoon egg substitute
- 1 tablespoon Red Star active dry yeast or 1 tablespoon other active dry yeast

Liquids:

- 4 egg whites

- 4 tablespoons canola oil

- 1 teaspoon cider vinegar

- 1 1/4 cups water

Directions:

1. In a medium-sized bowl, measure all of the dry ingredients.

2. Stir or whisk well.

3. Combine liquids and mix well.

Large Bread Machine method:

4. Transfer wet and dry ingredients and yeast to baking pan of bread machine in the order suggested by the manufacturer.

5. Press start.

6. Help mix dough during kneading cycle; Mixture will be very thick.

7. Use one rise and one knead cycle if machine is programmable.

8. Remove upon completion of baking cycle.

Oven method: Preheat oven to 375°F.

9. Lightly oil a 9-x-5-inch loaf pan.

10. Add yeast to mix and beat in liquids.

11. Beat 2 minutes

12. Scrape into loaf pan, cover with plastic wrap, and let rise to the top of the pan.

13. Bake 40-45 minutes or until lightly browned.

14. Cool on a wire rack before slicing.

Healthy Squash Bread

http://www.rachaelray.com/recipe.php?recipe_id=41
48

Serves 10

Ingredients

- Shortening, spray, or butter, for greasing the bread loaf pan (your choice based on your dairy tolerances)

- 1 1/2 cups whole wheat/white flour blend (you can use all white)

- 1/2 teaspoon salt

- 1 teaspoon baking soda

- 1/2 teaspoon each cinnamon, nutmeg and allspice *or* ground cloves

- 1 cup brown rice syrup

- 1 cup cooked, pureed winter squash such as Red Kuri, Acorn, Butternut, Pumpkin or Kabocha

- 1/2 cup extra virgin olive oil (EVOO)

- 2 eggs, organic if available

- 1/4 cup water

- 1/2 cup of chopped walnuts *or* pecans

Directions

1. Pre-heat the oven to 350°F. Butter a bread loaf pan.

2. Mix the dry ingredients into one bowl and thoroughly stir, even sift if you are feeling ambitious.

3. In a separate bowl, take the cooked squash and either whisk by hand or use a hand mixer to puree and fluff it up.

4. Then add the rice syrup and EVOO and thoroughly blend.

5. Separately, whisk the eggs together, then add to the squash and mix well.

6. Add water and then gradually add the dry ingredients, but blend by hand with a wooden spoon or spatula, not the mixer, as you do not want to over mix.

7. Add the nuts and stir again.

8. Pour the batter into the pan and bake until cooked through, about 70 minutes oven.

9. You can stick a fork or a toothpick in the center to test, but when you press the middle with your fingers, it should spring back, not indent.

10. Allow the bread to cool for 10 minutes in the pan, then turn it out onto a cooling rack and allow it to cool more.

11. Slice when you're hungry and top with apple spread or honey – or nothing at all!

12. To store, wrap in foil. You can freeze this, too.

Soups

Slow-Cooker Chicken Tortilla Soup

http://allrecipes.com/recipe/slow-cooker-chicken-tortilla-soup/detail.aspx

Yields: 8 servings

Ingredients:

- 1 pound shredded, cooked chicken
- 1 (15-ounce) can whole peeled tomatoes, mashed
- 1 (10-ounce) can enchilada sauce
- 1 medium chopped onion
- 1 (4-ounce) can chopped green Chile peppers
- 2 cloves garlic, minced
- 2 cups water
- 1 teaspoon cumin
- 1 teaspoon chili powder

- 1 teaspoon salt

- ¼ teaspoon black pepper

- 1 bay leaf

- 1 (10-ounce) package frozen corn

- 1 teaspoon chopped cilantro

- 7 corn tortillas

- Vegetable oil

Directions:

1. Place chicken, tomatoes, enchilada sauce, onion, green chilies, and garlic into a slow cooker.

2. Pour in water and chicken broth, and season with cumin, chili powder, salt, pepper, and bay leaf.

3. Stir in corn and cilantro. Cover, and cook on Low setting for 6 to 8 hours or on High setting for 3 to 4 hours.

4. Preheat oven to 400 degrees F (200 degrees C).

5. Lightly brush both sides of tortillas with oil. Cut tortillas into strips, then spread on a baking sheet.

6. Bake in preheated oven until crisp, about 10 to 15 minutes. To serve, sprinkle tortilla strips over soup.

Creamy Butternut Squash Soup

http://silk.com/recipes/creamy-butternut-squash-soup

Ingredients

- 1 1/2 lbs butternut squash
- 2 Tbsp olive oil
- 1 large onion, cut into large dice
- 1 Tbsp margarine (or butter)
- 1 pinch sugar
- 3 large garlic cloves, sliced
- 1 1/2 tsp cinnamon
- 1 tsp ground ginger
- 1/4 tsp ground cloves
- 1/8 tsp cayenne pepper
- 3 cups chicken broth
- 1 1/2 cups Silk Original soymilk
- Salt and freshly ground pepper, to taste

Directions

1. Cut the squash in half and remove the seeds. Lightly drizzle with olive oil and roast in a 400° F oven, cut side down, for 45 minutes. Cool, then remove skin and cut squash into 1-inch chunks.

2. Heat oil over medium-high heat in a large sauté pan until it's hot and shimmery.

3. Add butternut squash, then onion to the pan. Sauté, stirring very little at first, then more frequently, until squash starts to turn golden brown, 7 to 8 minutes.

4. Reduce heat to low and add margarine (or butter), sugar and garlic; continue cooking until all vegetables are a rich spotty caramel color, about 10 minutes longer.

5. Add cinnamon, ginger, cloves and cayenne pepper; continue to sauté until fragrant, 30 seconds to 1 minute longer.

6. Add broth and bring to a simmer over medium-high heat. Reduce heat to low and simmer, partially covered, for another 10 minutes.

7. Using a blender, purée until very smooth, 30 seconds to 1 minute. Vent the blender by removing the center of the lid or lifting one edge of the lid. Cover the top of the blender with a kitchen towel to prevent splatter. Pour the mixture into a soup pot.

8. Pour a bit more Silk into the blender and blend for a few seconds to remove excess soup from the blender. Pour the remainder into pot.

9. Begin to add Silk Original soymilk so the mixture reaches a soup consistency, yet remains thick enough to float garnish. Add salt and pepper to taste.

10. Heat through and ladle into bowls. It's lovely with sliced apple, a drizzle of sour cream, chopped walnuts, or a scoop of Greek yogurt and a sprinkle of cinnamon on top.

Pumpkin Soup

For best results, use a non-dairy milk alternative that contains carrageenan, which will help keep the liquid stabilized during heating.

Serves 4 to 6

Prep Time: 20 minutes

Cook Time: 20 minutes

Total Time: 40 minutes

Ingredients:

- 1 T. olive oil
- 1 cup finely chopped onion
- 1 clove garlic, finely chopped
- 1 medium-sized leek, white parts only, chopped
- 1 cup chopped apple or pear
- 3 T. sugar
- ¾ t. ground cinnamon
- ½ t. ground ginger
- ¼ t. ground nutmeg
- ½ t. salt, plus more to taste

- 1 15-ounce can low-sodium vegetable broth

- 2 cups water

- 2 15-ounce cans pumpkin puree

- ½ cup coconut milk

- ½ cup almond milk or soymilk (see Head Note)

- Pepper, to taste

- Cayenne, for garnishing

- Fresh herbs, such as dill or parsley, for garnishing

Directions

1. In a medium-large stock pot (3-5 quarts), heat the olive oil over medium-high heat. Add the onion and garlic, and cook for 3-4 minutes, or until the onion is translucent.

2. Add the leek, apple, sugar, spices and salt, and cook for 1-2 minutes, stirring constantly, until the leek is softened. Add the vegetable broth and water. Bring the mixture to a boil and then turn down to a simmer for about 15-20 minutes, or until the apple pieces are very tender.

3. Stir in the pumpkin puree. Working in batches, puree the mixture in a blender until smooth, adding a bit of the coconut milk and almond milk to each batch until all has been added.

4. Return the soup to the pot and heat over low heat, stirring constantly, to desired temperature. Add salt and pepper to taste. Garnish with a sprinkle of cayenne pepper and fresh herbs or your choice.

Spicy Tomato Soup Recipe

http://dairyfreecooking.about.com/od/soupschiliste
ws/r/Spicy_Tomato_Soup_Recipe.htm

Serves 4

Ingredients:

- 1 T. olive oil
- 1 large onion
- 4 large cloves garlic, finely chopped
- 1 large carrot, finely chopped
- 1 t. dried thyme
- 1/2 t. ground red pepper
- 1/4 t. cayenne
- 2 28-ounce cans whole peeled tomatoes in juice
- 1 cup low-sodium vegetable stock
- 2 cups plain soy milk
- 1 t. sugar
- Salt and pepper, to taste
- Parsley, for garnishing (optional)

Directions

1. In a large saucepan over medium-high heat, heat the olive oil, adding the onion, garlic, and carrot once hot.

2. Add the thyme, red pepper and cayenne, and cook for 5-6 minutes, stirring often, or until the onion is fragrant and the carrot is soft.

3. Add the tomatoes with juice and broth, bring to a simmer and cook, uncovered for 20-25 minutes.

4. Working in batches, puree the soup in a food processor or blender.

5. Return the pureed soup to the pot, add the soy milk and sugar, and cook until desired heat and consistency.

6. Add salt and pepper to taste. Serve hot, garnishing with parsley if desired.

Ginger-Soy Carrot Soup

http://www.rachaelray.com/recipe.php?recipe_id=37
05

Serves 4

Ingredients

- 2 tablespoons extra virgin olive oil (EVOO) *or* vegetable oil
- 1 large onion, chopped
- 3-4 cloves garlic, chopped
- 1 1-inch piece of ginger root, grated *or* finely chopped
- 1 chili pepper, seeded and chopped
- 2 pounds carrots, peeled and sliced *or* chopped
- 1/4 cup Tamari (dark soy sauce)
- 4 cups chicken stock (32 ounces)
- 1 cup water
- Salt and freshly ground black pepper
- Toasted sesame oil, for garnish
- 4 large eggs, fried (optional)

- Finely chopped chives or scallions, for garnish

- Toasted sesame rolls, for dunking

Directions

1. Heat the EVOO in large Dutch oven over medium-high heat.

2. Add the onion, garlic, ginger and chili pepper and sweat them out a few minutes.

3. Stir in the carrots and Tamari, then cover the pot and cook for 7-8 minutes.

4. Add the stock and bring to a boil. Reduce the heat and simmer the soup until the carrots are tender.

5. Puree as smooth or chunky as you like with hand blender or in a food processor, in batches. Season the soup with salt and pepper, to taste.

6. Cool completely and store in the refrigerator for a make-ahead meal.

7. Reheat, in a covered pot, over medium heat and serve in shallow bowls with a fried egg on top, cooked to your liking.

8. Garnish each serving with chives or scallions and a drizzle of toasted sesame oil on top. Pass the toasted sesame rolls at the table, for dunking.

Creamy Tomato Soup

http://silk.com/recipes/creamy-tomato-soup

Serves 4

- 1 Tbsp olive oil
- 1/2 medium onion, diced
- 1-2 cloves garlic, chopped
- 1 tsp salt
- 1 (28-oz) can whole tomatoes, undrained
- 1 cup vegetable broth
- 1 bay leaf
- 1/4 cup chopped fresh basil
- 1 tsp fresh thyme or 1/2 tsp dried thyme
- 1 cup Silk Original soymilk
- 1/4 cup Silk Original Creamer
- Fresh ground pepper

Directions

1. Heat olive oil over medium-low heat in a 4-quart stockpot.

2. Add the onion and sauté for 3-4 minutes.

3. Add the garlic and sauté an additional 3 minutes.

4. Add the salt, whole tomatoes with juice, vegetable broth, bay leaf, basil and thyme. Bring to a simmer and cook for 15 minutes, stirring occasionally to crush the tomatoes.

5. Remove the bay leaf; add Silk, Silk Creamer and a few grinds of fresh pepper.

6. Purée soup in 2 batches in a blender until smooth and creamy (use caution when blending hot soup).

7. Adjust salt and pepper to taste.

8. Return soup to pot, heat gently and serve

Lemongrass and Ginger Egg Drop Soup with Rainbow Chard

http://www.rachaelray.com/recipe.php?recipe_id=39

55

Serves 4

Ingredients

- 4 cups chicken stock (32 ounces)

- 2 cups water

- A few stems of lemongrass, cut into 3-inch lengths

- 1 large clove garlic, crushed

- 1 chili pepper, split

- 1 3-4-inch piece of fresh ginger root, divided

- 2 extra-large eggs

- 4 scallions, thinly sliced on an angle

- 2 cups rainbow chard, thinly shredded and packed

Directions

1. In a saucepot, add the stock, water, lemongrass, garlic, chili pepper and a couple inches of thick-sliced ginger.

2. Bring to a boil; reduce the heat to simmer and cover, steeping the flavor into the broth for 5-6 minutes.

   Strain the broth or skim out the flavorings with a slotted spoon.

3. Reduce the heat to low and peel and slice the remaining 1 inch of ginger into thin matchsticks and stir into the clear broth.

4. Beat the eggs, then swirl them slowly into the broth to create egg ribbons.

5. Add the scallions and wilt in the chard.

6. Remove from the heat and immediately serve in bowls.

Vegetable Posole (Mexican soup)

http://www.rachaelray.com/recipe.php?recipe_id=44 94

Serves 4-6

Ingredients

For the salsa verde:

- 2 large poblano peppers *or* 3 green New Mexican chili peppers

- 2 tablespoons corn oil *or* vegetable oil

- 1 onion, chopped

- 3-4 cloves garlic, chopped

- 6-7 medium tomatillos, paper husk removed and chopped

- 1 teaspoon cumin (1/3 palmful)

- 1 teaspoon coriander (1/3 palmful)

- Salt and pepper

- Juice of 1 lime

- 1 tablespoon honey

For the posole:

- About 3 tablespoons corn oil *or* vegetable oil

- 1 pound mixed mushrooms, chopped *or* thinly sliced

- Salt and pepper

- 1 1/2 teaspoons cumin (half a palmful)

- 1 1/2 teaspoons ground coriander (half a palmful)

- 1 1/2 teaspoons Mexican oregano (half a palmful), lightly crushed

- 1 teaspoon epazote (1/3 palmful), lightly crushed (optional)

- 1/2 bottle Mexican beer

- 2 cups homemade *or* store-bought salsa verde

- 2 cans hominy (14 ounces each can), drained

- 3 cups vegetable stock

- Cilantro leaves and thinly sliced scallions *or* chopped raw red onion, for garnish

Directions

1. To make the salsa verde, char the peppers over an open flame or under a hot broiler. Place the fully charred peppers in a bowl and cover with plastic wrap until cool. Peel, seed and reserve.

2. Heat the oil, about 2 tablespoons, in a skillet over medium-high heat. Add the onion and garlic and stir for a few minutes.

3. Add the tomatillos, cumin, coriander, salt and pepper and cook for 10 minutes more, until a sauce forms and thickens.

4. Add the mixture to a food processor or blender with the lime juice and honey. Process until fairly smooth.

5. For the posole, heat the oil, about 3 tablespoons, in a soup pot or Dutch oven over medium-high heat.

6. Add the mushrooms and brown well, 15 minutes.

7. Season with salt and pepper, cumin, coriander, oregano, epazote, if using, and stir for a minute more.

8. Deglaze with the beer. Add the salsa, hominy and stock, and simmer over low heat until ready to serve.

9. Serve in shallow bowls topped with the garnishes and charred tortillas on side.

Entrees & Sides

Non-Dairy/Lactose-Free/Vegan "cheese"

http://www.food.com/recipe/non-dairy-lactose-free-vegan-cheese-164469

Yields: 1 Serving

Ingredients

- 1 cup nutritional yeast flakes

- 1/3 cup white flour

- 3 tablespoons cornstarch

- 1 1/2 teaspoons salt

- 2 cups water

- 1/3 cup margarine

Directions

1. Mix dry ingredients in a saucepan. Gradually add water, making a smooth paste and then thin with the remaining water.

2. Place on heat and stir constantly until it thickens and bubbles. Let it bubble up for about 30 seconds and remove from heat. Whip in the margarine.

3. Good on pizza, casseroles, open-faced tomato sandwiches, grilled cheese sandwiches, macaroni and cheese, and enchiladas.

Lactose-Free Indian Curry

http://www.food.com/recipe/lactose-free-indian-curry-479439

Yields: 4 Servings

Ingredients

- 1 tablespoon olive oil

- 4 chicken drumsticks, deboned and cubed

- 1 cup soy yogurt, plain

- 3 whole allspice

- 2 teaspoons gingerroot, grated

- 2 teaspoons curry

- 1 teaspoon red pepper flakes

- 1 teaspoon cumin

- 1/2 cup water

- 1 tablespoon cornstarch

Directions

1. Heat olive oil, in a skillet, on medium high heat. Once hot, brown the drumstick meat in it, until it's properly cooked, about 5 minutes.

2. In a small bowl mix the plain soy yogurt with the seasonings, then slowly add it to the skillet, making sure the chicken is properly coated in it, as it is cooking. Stir occasionally for 3 minutes.

3. In another small bowl, mix water and cornstarch, until there it is smooth and there are no lumps. Add this to the chicken mixture, stirring occasionally for about 5 minutes or until sauce thickens.

4. Serve warm and over basmati rice.

Butternut Squash Carrot Avocado Almond Salad (gluten- and lactose-free)

http://www.food.com/recipe/butternut-squash-carrot-avo-almond-salad-gluten-lactose-free-330873

Yields: 1 Serving

Ingredients

- 2 cups green leaf lettuce (washed)
- 1/2 cup butternut squash (Roasted and mashed—temp. should be cold)
- 1/4 avocado (sliced)
- 1/2 cup carrot (grated)
- 1/4 cup natural almonds (chopped)
- 1 tablespoon olive oil (virgin)
- 4 tablespoons white balsamic vinegar

Directions:

1. Roast butternut squash for approximately 1 hour at 400°F

2. Spoon out mashy bits in middle and store until ready to make recipe. Do not use oil. Discard the skin and other hard bits.

3. Combine cold squash with lettuce and gently mix together.

4. Add avocado, carrot, and almonds.

5. Toss olive oil into salad.

6. Add vinegar and serve

Grilled Mediterranean Chicken (or Tofu) and Grape Skewers

http://www.godairyfree.org/recipes/grilled-mediterranean-skewer-recipe

Yields: 6 servings

Serving Size: 2 skewers

Ingredients

- 1/4 cup + 2 tablespoons extra virgin olive oil, divided

- 2 cloves garlic, fresh minced

- 1/2 teaspoon red chili flakes, crushed

- 1 tablespoon oregano, fresh minced

- 1 tablespoon rosemary, fresh minced

- 1 teaspoon lemon zest

- 1 pound chicken breast, boneless and skinless, cut into 3/4-inch cubes [can alternately use extra-firm, pressed tofu or tempeh cut into cubes]

- 1-3/4 cups California green seedless grapes

- 1/2 teaspoon salt

- 2 tablespoons extra virgin olive oil

- 1 tablespoon lemon juice, fresh

Directions:

1. In small bowl, whisk the 1/4 cup of olive oil, garlic, chili flakes, oregano, rosemary and lemon zest.

2. Alternately thread the chicken pieces and grapes onto 12 skewers (if using wooden skewers, make sure they have been adequately soaked).

3. Place the skewers into a baking dish or pan large enough to hold them, and pour the marinade over top, making sure to generously coating each skewer.

4. Let the skewers marinate for 4 to 24 hours.

5. Remove skewers from marinade and let excess oil drip off.

6. Season the skewers with the salt.

7. Grill until the chicken is cooked through, about 3 to 5 minutes on each side.

8. Arrange the skewers on a serving platter and drizzle with the remaining 2 tablespoons of olive oil and the lemon juice.

Notes:

For vegan and vegetarian, this marinade goes very nicely with tofu, or you may prefer it with something "meatier" like tempeh.

This recipe is optionally vegan, optionally vegetarian, dairy free, egg free, gluten free, nut free, peanut free, soy free (though not with the vegan options), wheat free, and sugar free.

1. Combine the eggs and the sliced wheat bread cubes. Add the turkey broth to this mixture and sprinkle the spices. If the mixture is too thick or crumbly, add more broth. However, do not add too much broth as this will make the mixture too light and mushy. You wouldn't want the filling to be too mushy as this will affect the flavor.

2. Add the first mixture (the one with onions) and blend the ingredients well.

3. Place the finished mixture into a pre-sprayed baking dish and cover with foil. Add a bit of soy-based margarine on top before baking for 20 minutes (add a parchment cover). After cooking, remove the parchment and cook for another half hour. Serve hot.

Cheese Pizza with Basil Leaves

http://www.rachaelray.com/recipe.php?recipe_id=45 57

Serves 4-6

Ingredients

- 1 pound frozen pizza dough, defrosted

- 1/4 cup flour

- 3 tablespoons olive oil, divided, plus extra for garnish

- 2 tablespoons cornmeal

- 2 cloves garlic, minced

- Salt and pepper

- 1 cup whole, peeled tomatoes, canned

- 1 cup fresh basil leaves

- 1 tablespoon dried oregano

- 1 cup shredded mozzarella-style Daiya brand cheese

- Chili flakes, for garnish

- Salt and pepper

Directions

1. Preheat the oven to 450°F.

2. Roll the dough out as thinly as possible. If you have a 14-inch round pizza stone or pan, the dough should reach just over the edges of the pan. If you are using a baking sheet, roll the dough in a rectangle shape.

3. Lightly oil the pan. Spread out the cornmeal, then lay the dough on the pan. Roll in the edges of the dough to prevent burning.

4. Drizzle the dough with 2 tablespoons of the olive oil and spread it evenly over the dough with your fingers.

5. Spread the minced garlic and season with 1/8 teaspoon salt and 1/8 teaspoon black pepper.

6. Break up the tomatoes into smaller pieces and spread them over the dough.

7. Slice with a pizza cutter and garnish with chili flakes and olive oil followed by the basil leaves, oregano and shredded cheese.

8. Top the pizza with the remaining 1 tablespoon olive oil and a dash of salt. Brush the rolled edges with a little cold water.

9. Put the pizza in the oven and bake for 15 minutes.

10. If it's not done, rotate the pan and check again in 5 minutes. When the pizza is done, the cheese should just be starting to brown.

Mexican Fiesta Dairy-Free or Vegan Pizza

http://www.godairyfree.org/recipes/entrees/dairy-free-Mexican-vegan-pizza

Prep Time: 10 minutes

Cook Time: 18 minutes

Total Time: 28 minutes

Yield: 4 servings /1 pizza

Ingredients

- 1 medium to large whole wheat vegan or gluten-free flatbread or pre-made pizza shell
- 1/2 cup prepared vegan pizza sauce
- 1/2 cup ground beef or vegan "beef" alternative
- 3/4 cup Vegan Mexican Style Shreds
- 1/4 red bell pepper, diced
- 1/4 green bell pepper, diced
- 1/4 yellow bell pepper, diced
- Fresh cilantro

Directions

1. Preheat the oven to 425°F.

2. Spray a large cookie sheet or sheet pan with a spritz of vegetable oil spray. Place the flatbread on the sheet.

3. Top the flatbread with the pizza sauce and spread evenly. Distribute the ground "beef" alternative over the sauce evenly, followed by the Vegan Mexican Style Shreds. Add all peppers, spreading evenly over the surface of the Shreds.

4. Place sheet pan in the oven and bake for 18 minutes, or until the Vegan Shreds are melted and light brown.

5. Remove, and top with cilantro while still hot. Let cool for 5 minutes to allow ingredients to set. Slice into wedges and serve

BBQ Pork for Sandwiches—Slow Cooker Pulled Pork

http://allrecipes.com/recipe/bbq-pork-for-sandwiches/detail.aspx

Yields: 12 servings

Ingredients

- 1 (14-ounce) can beef broth

- 3 pounds boneless pork ribs

- 1 (18-ounce) bottle barbeque sauce

Directions:

1. Pour can of beef broth into slow cooker, and add boneless pork ribs. Cook on high heat for 4 hours or until meat shreds easily. Remove meat, and shred with two forks.

2. Preheat oven to 350 degrees F (175 degrees C). Transfer the shredded pork to a Dutch oven or iron skillet, and stir in barbeque sauce.

3. Bake in the preheated oven for 30 minutes, or until heated through.

4. Mix the rice in the pan so the oil is evenly distributed throughout. The rice will also become a little crisp. This should take about 4 minutes of constant stirring.

5. Add 4 ounces of wine to the slightly crispy rice mixture. Continue mixing and stirring the rice so the wine will be absorbed more quickly. This phase of the cooking process will be completed once the wine has been absorbed by the rice.

6. Add a 3/4th cup of the chicken broth to the rice. Again, continue mixing the rice until everything has been absorbed. Continue adding the chicken broth until all of the broth has been absorbed. Cook the rice for an additional 20 minutes.

7. When the rice is finally cooked, it's time to add the cooked shrimp and chopped spinach. Soy margarine can be added as a final flavoring to the dish. Don't forget to grind some pepper on the risotto before serving warm.

Lactose-Free Cheesy French Fries

http://dairyfreecooking.about.com/od/potatoes /r/CheesyFries.htm

These savory potato wedges are easy to prepare and can be frozen and reheated for a quick snack or bistro-style side dish. The cheese sauce is best right after it is made, but to save time, make a mix of the dry ingredients and store it in an airtight container in your pantry.

Serves 4

Prep Time: 15 minutes

Cook Time: 35 minutes

Total Time: 50 minutes

Ingredients:

- 4 large gold potatoes, scrubbed and cut into wedges

- 2 T olive oil

- 1/3 cup nutritional yeast

- 1 t. tumeric

- 1 cup unsweetened soymilk (not non-fat)

- 2 T. tahini

- 1/4 cup vegetable broth powder

- 1 T. prepared mustard

- Salt and pepper, to taste

Directions

1. Preheat the oven to 400 F. Lightly oil a large baking sheet.

2. Place the potato wedges in a single layer on the prepared sheet. Brush with some of the oil and generously salt and pepper.

3. Bake for about 35 to 40 minutes, flipping half-way through or when the fries begin to brown, brushing with oil as needed.

4. Meanwhile, prepare the cheese sauce. Combine the nutritional yeast and tumeric in a small dish and set aside.

5. In a small sauce pan over medium-low heat, heat the soymilk and tahini. When just warm, add the nutritional yeast mixture, stirring until well combined. Add the vegetable broth powder, stirring well until dissolved.

6. Add the prepared mustard and cook until desired consistency, keeping in mind that the sauce will thicken slightly as it begins to cool. Salt and pepper to taste.

7. Pour cheesy sauce over French fries and serve hot.

Creamy Polenta with Sautéed Leafy Greens

http://www.rachaelray.com/recipe.php?recipe_id=45 64

Serves 4

Ingredients

For the polenta:
- 3 cups water
- A pinch of salt
- 1 cup polenta grains

For the cream sauce:
- 3/4 cup raw cashews, soaked in water for 1 hour
- 4 tablespoons olive oil, divided
- 2 cloves garlic, minced
- 3 tablespoons lemon juice
- 1 teaspoon salt
- 3/4 cup white beans
- 1 cup water

For the greens:

- 3 tablespoons olive oil

- 4 cups spinach, kale, collard greens *or* chard, stemmed and coarsely chopped

- Salt and pepper

Directions

1. In a medium size saucepan, bring 3 cups of water to a boil with a pinch of salt.

2. Slowly stir in the polenta. Reduce the heat to low and simmer gently for 30 minutes, stirring often to prevent the polenta from sticking.

3. Heat a pan over low heat and add the olive oil, followed by the garlic. Cook until the garlic begins to soften, stirring often. Cool to room temperature.

4. Strain the cashews. Place the cashews in a blender with the garlic and its cooking oil, lemon juice, salt, white beans and water and blend until smooth. With the blender still going, slowly pour in the remaining 2 tablespoons oil.

5. When the polenta is almost done, cook the greens.

6. Heat a sauté pan and add the olive oil, then the greens.

7. Cook over medium heat for 5 minutes, stirring often, until tender. Season with salt.

8. Take the polenta off the heat and stir in the cream sauce. Season, to taste. Serve topped with greens and a few grinds of fresh pepper.

Yummy Honey Chicken Kabobs

http://allrecipes.com/recipe/yummy-honey-chicken-kabobs/detail.aspx

Yields: 12 servings

Ingredients

- ¼ cup vegetable oil
- 1/3 cup honey
- 1/3 cup soy sauce
- ¼ cup teaspoon ground black pepper
- 8 skinless, boneless chick breast halves—cut into 1 inch cubes
- 2 cloves garlic
- 5 small onions—cut into 2-inch pieces
- 2 red bell peppers—cut into 2-inch pieces
- skewers

Directions

1. In a large bowl, whisk together oil, honey, soy sauce, and pepper. Before adding chicken, reserve a small amount of marinade to brush onto kabobs while cooking.

2. Place the chicken, garlic, onions and peppers in the bowl, and marinate in the refrigerator at least 2 hours (the longer the better).

3. Preheat the grill for high heat.

4. Drain marinade from the chicken and vegetables, and discard marinade.

5. Thread chicken and vegetables alternately onto the skewers.

6. Lightly oil the grill grate. Place the skewers on the grill. Cook for 12 to 15 minutes, until chicken juices run clear.

7. Turn and brush with reserved marinade frequently.

Grilled Asparagus

http://allrecipes.com/recipe/grilled-asparagus/detail.aspx

Yields: 4 servings

Ingredients

- 1 pound fresh asparagus spears, trimmed
- 1 tablespoon olive oil
- Salt and pepper to taste

Directions

1. Preheat grill for high heat.
2. Lightly coat the asparagus spears with olive oil. Season with salt and pepper to taste.
3. Grill over high heat for 2 to 3 minutes, or to desired tenderness.

Sesame Green Beans

http://allrecipes.com/recipe/sesame-green-beans/detail.aspx

Yields: 4 servings

Ingredients

- 1 tablespoon olive oil

- 1 tablespoon sesame seeds

- 1 pound fresh green beans, cut into 2-inch pieces

- ¼ cup chicken broth

- ¼ teaspoon salt

- Freshly ground black pepper to taste

Directions

1. Heat oil in a large skillet or wok over medium heat.

2. Add sesame seeds.

3. When seeds start to darken, stir in green beans.

4. Cook, stirring, until the beans turn bright green.

5. Pour in chicken broth, salt and pepper.

6. Cover and cook until beans are tender-crisp, about 10 minutes. Uncover, cook until liquid evaporates.

Easy Baked Salmon with Wilted Spinach and Strawberry Salsa

http://www.godairyfree.org/recipes/salmon-recipe-strawberry-salsa

Yields: 4 light meals

Ingredients:

- 4 (4-ounce) salmon fillets, skin removed

- 1 teaspoon lemon zest

- salt and pepper, to taste

- 1 pound strawberries, diced

- 2 kiwifruits, peeled and diced

- 1 cucumber, diced

- 1 jalapeño, seeded and minced

- 2 tablespoons chopped fresh mint leaves

- 2 tablespoons fresh lemon juice, divided

- 1 pound baby spinach leaves, rinsed but not dried

Directions:

1. Preheat your oven to 350°F.

2. Place the salmon on a baking sheet and sprinkle with lemon zest and a little salt and pepper.

3. Bake for 15 to 18 minutes or until cooked through.

4. Meanwhile, place the strawberries, kiwi, cucumber, jalapeño, mint and 1 tablespoon of the lemon juice in a medium bowl and toss until combined. Set aside.

5. Heat a large, high-sided skillet over medium heat. Add the spinach, with water still clinging to leaves, cover and cook 5 minutes or until wilted, stirring occasionally.

6. Stir in the remaining 1 tablespoon of lemon juice.

7. Divide the spinach among 4 plates, and top with the salmon and salsa and serve.

Sesame Pasta Chicken Salad

http://allrecipes.com/recipe/sesame-pasta-chicken-salad/detail.aspx

Yields: 10 servings

Ingredients

- ¼ cup sesame seeds
- 1 (16-ounce) package bow tie pasta
- ½ cup vegetable oil
- 1/3 cup light soy sauce
- 1/3 cup rice vinegar
- 1 teaspoon sesame oil
- 3 tablespoons white sugar
- ½ teaspoon ground ginger
- 14 teaspoon ground black pepper
- 3 cups shredded, cooked chicken breast meat
- ½ cup chopped fresh cilantro
- 1/3 cup chopped green onion

Directions

1. Heat a skillet over medium-high heat. Add sesame seeds, and cook stirring frequently until lightly toasted. Remove from heat, and set aside.

2. Bring a large pot of lightly salted water to a boil. Add pasta, and cook for 8 to 10 minutes, or until al dente. Drain pasta, and rinse under cold water until cool. Transfer to a large bowl.

3. In a jar with a tight-fitting lid, combine vegetable oil, soy sauce, vinegar, sesame oil, sugar, sesame seeds, ginger, and pepper. Shake well.

4. Pour sesame dressing over pasta, and toss to coat evenly.

5. Gently mix in chicken, cilantro, and green onions.

Pork Chops Smothered with Peppers and Onions

http://www.rachaelray.com/recipe.php?recipe_id=44
66

Serves 4

Ingredients

- 4 bone-in pork chops, 1 1/2-inches thick, at room temperature
- Kosher salt and freshly ground black pepper
- 3 tablespoons extra virgin olive oil (EVOO), divided
- 4 cloves garlic
- 1 large onion
- 1-2 cubanelle peppers
- 1 red bell pepper, seeded
- 1 red chili pepper
- 1 teaspoon fennel seed
- 2 tablespoons tomato paste
- 1/2 cup dry white wine *or* red wine

- 1 1/2 cups chicken stock

Directions

1. Pre-heat the oven to 400°F.

2. Sprinkle the chops with liberal amounts of salt and black pepper.

3. Heat 2 tablespoons of the EVOO in a large skillet over medium-high to high heat. When the EVOO begins to smoke, add the chops and brown on both sides, 3-4 minutes per side.

4. While the chops cook, slice the garlic, onion and peppers.

5. Remove the chops from the skillet and add the remaining tablespoon EVOO. Then add the fennel seed, garlic, onion and peppers and toss to soften, 5 minutes.

6. Next, add the tomato paste and stir, 1 minute.

7. Deglaze the pan with the wine; add the stock and stir. Nestle the pork into the pan and move the peppers and onions on top of the meat.

8. Place in the oven and roast to an internal temperature of 165°F, about 10 minutes.

Pork Stew with Fennel and Apricots

http://www.rachaelray.com/recipe.php?recipe_id=4499

Serves 4

Ingredients

- 3 tablespoons extra virgin olive oil (EVOO), divided
- 1 boneless pork butt (1 1/2 pounds), cut into 2-inch pieces
- Salt and pepper
- 1 medium red onion, halved and thinly sliced
- 3 cloves garlic, sliced
- 1 sprig oregano
- 2 anchovy fillets
- 1 large bulb fennel, stems and fronds trimmed off and bulb quartered lengthwise
- 3/4 cup dried apricots (about 4 ounces)

Directions

1. In a 6-quart Dutch oven, heat 2 tablespoons EVOO over medium heat. Working in batches, add the pork, season with salt and pepper and brown on all sides, about 5 minutes per batch. Transfer to a bowl.

2. Pour off the fat from the pan. Add the onion, garlic, oregano, anchovies and the remaining tablespoon EVOO to the pan and season with salt and pepper.

3. Cover and cook over low heat, stirring occasionally, until softened, 8-10 minutes.

4. Add 2 cups water and bring to a boil over medium-high heat, stirring to scrape up any browned bits from the bottom of the pan.

5. Add the pork, fennel bulb and stems and the apricots; season again and press a piece of parchment on top.
   Cover and cook over low heat until the meat is very tender, about 1 1/2 hours.

6. Discard the fennel stems, then ladle the stew into large, shallow bowls and garnish with fennel fronds.

Grilled Salmon

http://allrecipes.com/recipe/grilled-salmon-i/detail.aspx

Yields: 6 servings

Ingredients:

- 1 ½ pounds salmon fillets
- Lemon pepper to taste
- Garlic powder to taste
- Salt to taste
- 1/3 cup soy sauce
- 1/3 cup brown sugar
- 1/3 cup water
- ¼ cup vegetable oil

Directions

1. Season salmon fillets with lemon pepper, garlic powder, and salt.

2. In a small bowl, stir together soy sauce, brown sugar, water, and vegetable oil until sugar is dissolved.

3. Place fish in a large resealable plastic bag with the soy sauce mixture, seal, and turn to coat. Refrigerate for at least 2 hours.

4. Preheat grill for medium heat.

5. Lightly oil grill grate. Place salmon on the preheated grill, and discard marinade. Cook salmon for 6 to 8 minutes per side, or until the fish flakes easily with a fork.

Pot Roast

http://www.drgourmet.com/recipes/maincourse/beef/potroast.shtml

Servings = 6 | Serving size =6 ounces beef with potatoes and veggies

Cooking Time = 4 hours

This recipe can be multiplied by 2, 3.

This recipe makes great leftovers. There will be two ounces beef left over after the five servings - just enough for a sandwich for lunch! Save a little gravy to go on it.

Ingredients

- 2 tsp olive oil

- 2 lbs bottom round (trimmed of excess fat)

- 1 cup water

- 2 bay leaves

- 1 Tbsp dried sage

- 1 tsp salt

- Fresh ground black pepper (to taste)

- 2 medium onions (cut into wedges)

- 2 lbs small red potatoes (cut into large chunks)

- 1 lb carrots (peeled and thickly sliced)

Directions

1. Preheat the oven to 225°F.

2. Place the oil in a Dutch oven or medium stock pot over medium high heat. When the oil is hot, add the bottom round to the pot.

3. Sear the meat on each side for about 2 minutes per side.

4. Add the water and remove from heat. Add the bay leaves, sage, salt, pepper and onion and stir.

5. Cover the pot and place in the oven. Let roast for 3 hours.

6. Remove the pan from the oven (be careful when taking the lid off).

7. Remove about half of the onions and liquid and place in a blender or food processor.

8. Puree until smooth and set aside.

9. Add the potatoes and carrots to the pot. Return the pot to the oven for another 60 – 90 minutes.

10. Remove the roast from the oven and place the roast on a plate.

11. Add the pureed onions to the pot and stir well to thicken the gravy. Serve topped with gravy.

Chopped Nicoise Salad

http://www.drgourmet.com/recipes/salad/chopped nicoise.shtml

Servings = 2 | Serving size =about 3 cups

Cooking Time = 30 Minutes

This recipe can be multiplied by 2, 3, 4, 5, 6, 7, 8.

Once tossed together, this recipe does not make good leftovers. You could, however, refrigerate the ingredients the night before and put the salad together at the last minute.

Ingredients

- 1 quart water

- 2 large eggs

- 3 quarts water

- 12 ounces red potatoes (peeled and cut into small dice)

- 8 ounces green beans

- 2 Tbsp olive oil

- ½ lemon (juiced)

- 2 tsp honey

- 2 tsp coarse ground mustard

- 1 tsp fresh thyme leaves

- 1 clove garlic (minced)

- ¼ tsp salt

- Fresh ground black pepper to taste

- 12 grape tomatoes (halved)

- 10 large black olives (cut into slivers)

- 12 large leaves romaine lettuce (thinly sliced crosswise)

- 2 Tbps capers (drained)

- 1 can (6 ½ ounce low-sodium light tuna in water-- drained)

Directions

1. Place the 1 quart water in a sauce pan and bring to a boil. Place the eggs in the pot and cook for 3 minutes. Turn off the heat and let stand for 12 minutes. Remove and run under cool water. Peel the eggs and put in the refrigerator.

2. Place the water in a large stock pot over high heat.

3. Add the diced potatoes and add to the stock pot. Bring to a boil, then reduce heat until the water is simmering. Cook for about 10 minutes.

4. Remove the potatoes from the hot water (leave the water in the pot) and plunge them into ice water. Let cool, remove from the ice water, then place the potatoes in the refrigerator.

5. Add the green beans to the water in the pot and cook for about 5 – 7 minutes. Remove and plunge into ice water. Remove and place the green beans in the refrigerator.

6. Place the olive oil, lemon juice, honey, mustard, thyme, garlic, salt and pepper in a large bowl. Whisk until smooth. Place in the freezer for about 5 minutes to chill.

7. Remove the vinaigrette from the freezer and whisk. Add the tomatoes, olives, romaine and capers and toss well.

8. Coarsely chop the eggs and add them to the bowl.

9. Slice the green beans into 1 inch lengths and add them to the bowl along with the potatoes.

10. Add the tuna and toss until the salad is blended. Serve.

Grilled Halibut with Tangerines and Capers

http://www.drgourmet.com/recipes/maincourse/fish/halibuttangerine.shtml

Servings = 2 | Serving size = 4 ounces fish with topping

Cooking Time = 30 Minutes

This recipe can be multiplied by 2, 3, 4, 5, 6, 7, 8, 9, 10.

This recipe makes great leftovers as sandwiches.

Ingredients

- 1 small shallot (minced)

- 1 clove garlic (minced)

- 1 tangerine (peeled, seeded, and separated into sections)

- 1 Tbsp olive oil

- 2 tsp caper juice

- 2 tsp capers

- ¼ tsp salt

- 1 Tbsp cilantro leaves

- 2 four ounce halibut filets

- Spray-style olive oil

Directions:

- Combine the shallot, garlic, tangerine, olive oil, caper liquid, capers, salt, pepper and cilantro. Toss and then chill.

- When ready to cook, place a large non-stick skillet over high heat. Spray lightly with oil when the pan is hot and then add the halibut filets. Cook for about 6-8 minutes, then turn and cook for another 6-8 minutes.

- Serve over rice and top with the tangerine mixture.

Maple Sage Turkey Breast

http://www.drgourmet.com/recipes/maincourse/chicken/maplesageturkey.shtml

Servings = 8 | Serving size =4 ounces turkey breast

Cooking Time = 150 Minutes

This recipe makes great leftovers as sandwiches.

Ingredients:

- 1 3lb. bone-in turkey breast

- 1 large white onion (peeled and cut into eighths)

- 2 Tbsp fresh sages leaves

- ½ tsp peppercorns

- ½ tsp dried thyme leaves

- ½ cup maple syrup

- ½ cup low sodium chicken or vegetable broth

- ½ tsp salt

Directions

1. Preheat the oven to 325°F.

2. Rinse the whole turkey breast in cold water and pat dry.

3. Line a roasting pan with aluminum foil. Place the onion pieces in the bottom on top of the aluminum foil in a mound. Scatter the sage, thyme and peppercorns over the top of the onions.

4. Place the turkey breast on top of the onions (skin side up) and cover lightly with aluminum foil, then place the pan inside the preheated oven.

5. Roast for 30 minutes, then turn the roasting pan 180° in the oven (to make sure the turkey roasts evenly).

6. After another half hour remove the aluminum foil.

7. Top with 1/4 cup of the maple syrup and return the pan to the oven.

8. After another 30 to 45 minutes, baste the turkey with the juices from the bottom of the pan and add the other 1/4 cup maple syrup. If the skin is getting too crispy, you can put the foil back over the top.

9. Cook until the internal temperature of the breast meat is 160°F.
    Remove to a cutting board and allow to rest for at least 10 minutes before carving.

10. While the turkey is resting, skim the excess fat from the bottom of the roasting pan and discard.

11. Place the roasted onions, herbs and remaining liquid in a blender and puree until smooth.

12. Add up to 1/2 cup chicken stock to the desired thickness (it might take less, but if it is still not thin enough, use a little water - about a tablespoon at a time).

13. Reheat the sauce gently and serve over the sliced turkey.

Barbecue Shrimp Salad

http://www.drgourmet.com/recipes/salad/bbqshri
mpsalad.shtml

Servings = 4 | Serving size =1 1/2 cups salad

Cooking Time = 90 Minutes

This recipe can be multiplied by 2, 3, 4, 5.

This recipe makes great leftovers. Keep in the refrigerator
for no more than 48 hours.

Ingredients

- 2 cloves garlic (sliced)
- 1 small shallot (diced)
- 2 tsp paprika
- 1 tsp chili powder
- 1 Tbsp molasses
- ¼ tsp pure vanilla extract
- ½ tsp ground cumin
- ½ tsp salt
- ¼ tsp fresh ground black pepper
- 1 Tbsp grape seed or olive oil

- 1 lb large shrimp (peeled and deveined)

- Spray olive or grape seed oil

Directions

1. Combine the garlic, shallot, paprika, chili powder, molasses, vanilla extract, ground cumin, salt, pepper, grape seed oil and shrimp in a large zipper bag.

2. Toss the shrimp in the bag until well coated with the spices. This can be done up to 24 hours in advance and kept in the refrigerator. The shrimp will be best if they marinate for at least a few hours.

3. When you are ready to serve, preheat the oven to 400°F. Place a large non-stick skillet in the oven and after the oven is hot spray the hot pan lightly with oil.

4. Add the diced onions to the pan and return the skillet to the oven. Cook the onions for about 5, stir and cook for five more minutes in the oven.

5. Add the shrimp. Cook for about 7 - 10 minutes tossing the shrimp in the pan a couple of times.

6. Remove from the oven and place in a large bowl. Let the barbecued shrimp cool and then cover and chill for about an hour.

7. After the shrimp is cooled fold in the diced celery and mayonnaise and serve.

Curried Shrimp and Coconut Rice Salad

http://www.drgourmet.com/recipes/salad/curriedshrimp.shtml

Servings = 4 | Serving size =about 2 cups

Cooking Time = 90 Minutes

This recipe can be multiplied by 2, 3, 4.

This recipe can be divided by 2.

Cooking time includes chilling time. Refrigerated, this recipe keeps well for 24-36 hours only.

Ingredients

- 3 cups water

- 1 cup light coconut milk

- 1 cup brown jasmine rice

- 2 tsp olive oil

- 1 large shallot (minced)

- ½ tsp cinnamon

- 4 tsp curry powder

- ¼ tsp red pepper flakes

- 1 lb shrimp (peeled, deveined and halved lengthwise)

- 2 Tbsp peanut butter (no salt or sugar added)

- ¼ cup raisins

- 3 large ribs celery (diced)

- 1 cup frozen peas

- ½ tsp salt

Directions

1. Place the water and coconut milk in a medium pan over high heat. When the water boils add the rice. Reduce the heat to a simmer and boil slowly until all the water has evaporated.

2. When the rice is cooked place it in a large mixing bowl.

3. While the rice is cooking, place the oil in a large skillet over medium heat.

4. Add the minced shallot and cook for about 2 minutes. Stir frequently.

5. Add the cinnamon, curry powder and red pepper flakes. Cook for about 2 minutes and stir frequently.

6. Add the shrimp and cook for about 10 minutes until the shrimp are pink and just cooked through.

7. While the salad and rice are still warm, add the peanut butter and mix well.

8. Add the raisins, celery, peppers, peas and salt to the bowl and mix well. Chill well before serving.

Green Beans in Walnut Vinaigrette

http://www.drgourmet.com/recipes/salad/greenbea
nswalnutvin.shtml

Servings = 6 | Serving size =4 ounces green beans

Cooking Time = 30 Minutes

This recipe can be multiplied by 2.

This recipe keeps well but the beans will turn gray-green in the refrigerator.

Ingredients

- 2 Tbsp shallot

- 2 Tbsp fresh lemon juice

- ¼ cup red wine vinegar

- 2 Tbsp extra virgin olive oil

- 1 ounce pure walnut extract

- ¼ tsp salt

- 1 tsp granulated sugar

- 2 cup water

- 1 ½ lbs fresh green beans

Directions

1. Combine the shallot, lemon juice, vinegar and walnut extract in a mixing bowl.

2. Slowly add the oil while whisking to blend completely.

3. Add the sugar 1/4 tsp. at a time to adjust for acidity to taste.

4. Chill completely in freezer whisking occasionally so the dressing doesn't freeze.

5. Place the water in a medium stock pot and set a steamer basket inside the pot. Place the pot on the range over high heat. Steam the green beans until they turn bright green and are slightly tender. This will take 10 - 15 minutes. Toss the beans at about five minutes and again at ten minutes so they cook evenly.

6. Remove them from the heat and place in the cold vinaigrette immediately. Toss for about 2 minutes until coated well. Chill.

7. Serve as soon as chilled (this can be kept for days but the beans will slowly turn grey-green in the refrigerator.)

Mediterranean Corn Salad

http://www.drgourmet.com/recipes/extras/medcorn
salad.shtml

Servings = 2 | Serving size =about 2 cups

Cooking Time = 30 Minutes

This recipe can be multiplied by 2, 3, 4, 5, 6, 7, 8.

This recipe makes great leftovers. Cooking time does not
include chilling time.

Ingredients

- 2 ears fresh corn

- 4 large black olives (minced very finely)

- 1 small green bell pepper (finely diced)

- 1 small shallot (minced)

- 1 medium tomato (seeded and diced)

- 1/8 tsp salt

- Fresh ground pepper to taste

- 4 large leaves fresh basil (chiffonade)

- 1 tsp extra virgin olive oil

Directions

1. Preheat the oven to 325°F.

2. Peel the husks back from the corn and remove the silks. Rinse well and then fold the husks back around the corn. Wrap with aluminum foil.

3. Place the corn in the oven and roast for 25 minutes. Remove and let cool.

4. Shuck the corn from the cob and add it to a bowl with the olives, peppers, shallot, tomato, salt, pepper, basil and olive oil.

5. Fold together and chill.

Curried Lentil Salad with Lamb

http://www.drgourmet.com/recipes/salad/curriedlentillamb.shtml

Servings = 4 | Serving size =about 3 cups

Cooking Time = 30 Minutes

This recipe can be multiplied by 2, 3, 4, 5, 6, 7, 8.

This recipe makes great leftovers. Note that cooking time does not include chilling time.

Ingredients

- 3 ½ cups water

- 1 cup green lentils

- 2 tsp olive oil

- 12 ounces lamb shoulder or leg (cut into small cubes)

- 1 tsp ground cumin

- 1 tsp curry powder

- 4 Tbsp reduced fat mayonnaise

- ¾ tsp salt

- Fresh ground black pepper (to taste)

- 3 medium green onions (sliced crosswise)

- 2 ribs celery (diced)

- 1 small green bell pepper (diced)

- ¼ cup raw pistachios (shelled)

- 1/3 cup raisins

- 8 ounces fresh spinach leaves

Directions

1. Place the water in a large sauce pan over high heat. When it is boiling add the lentils. Cook about 20 minutes until tender.

2. Drain, rinse and put into the refrigerator to chill.

3. Place the olive oil in a large skillet over medium high heat. When the oil is hot, add the lamb cubes.

4. Cook, tossing frequently, for about ten minutes until well browned. Remove to a plate and place in the refrigerator to chill.

5. Mix the cumin, curry powder, mayonnaise, salt and pepper together until well blended, and place the dressing in the bowl with the lentils. Add the lamb and fold together until blended.

6. Add the green onions, carrots, celery, bell pepper, pistachios, raisins and spinach. Fold together until well blended.

7. Chill until ready to serve.

Citrus Vinaigrette

http://www.drgourmet.com/recipes/salad/citrusvin aigrette.shtml

Servings = 6 | Serving size =2 Tbsp. dressing

Cooking Time = 30 Minutes

This recipe can be multiplied by 2.

This vinaigrette keeps well for about 4 - 7 days.

Ingredients

- 1 clove garlic (peeled and crushed)
- 2 Tbsp extra virgin olive oil
- ¼ cup fresh lemon juice
- 5 Tbsp white wine vinegar
- 2 Tbsp honey
- ½ tsp ground dry mustard

Directions

Place garlic, olive oil, lemon juice, vinegar, honey and mustard in a blender and blend on high.

Crab, Avocado and Mango Salad

http://www.drgourmet.com/recipes/salad/crabavocadomango.shtml

Servings = 4 | Serving size =about 2 1/2 cups salad

Cooking Time = 30 Minutes

This recipe can be multiplied by 2, 3, 4, 5, 6, 7, 8

This recipe can be divided by 2

Cooking time does not include chilling time (although it's close). This recipe keeps well in the refrigerator for about 36 hours.

Ingredients

- 1 lb crabmeat (look for pasteurized)

- 1 large mango (peeled and diced)

- 1 medium avocado (peeled and diced)

- 1 lime (juiced)

- 1 small shallot (minced)

- ¼ tsp salt

- 1Tbsp olive oil

- Fresh ground pepper to taste

- 12 large leaves fresh basil (chiffonade)

Directions

1. Pick over the crabmeat carefully to remove any bits of shell.

2. Fold together the crabmeat, mango, lime juice, shallot, salt, pepper, olive oil and basil.

3. Chill.

Spinach Salad with Ginger Dressing and Sesame Chicken

http://www.drgourmet.com/recipes/salad/sesamec

hicken.shtml

Servings = 3 | Serving size =salad with 4 ounces chicken

Cooking Time = 45 Minutes

This recipe can be multiplied by 2,3.

This recipe makes great sandwiches the next day. Serve with 2 ounces brown bread and a tablespoon of Orange Marmalade.

Ingredients

- 2 Tbsp grape seed oil

- ¼ cup frozen orange juice concentrate (thawed)

- 1/8 tsp salt

- 1/8 tsp fresh ground black pepper

- 2 Tbsp crystallized ginger (minced)

- 1 tsp minced parsley

- 1 Tbsp minced chives

- 3 Tbsp slivered almonds

- 3 Tbsp black sesame seeds

- 3 four-ounce boneless chicken breasts (cut into one inch strips)

- 9 ounces baby spinach

- 1 fifteen-ounce can mandarin oranges (drained of all syrup)

- ½ small red onion (sliced as thinly as possible)

Directions

1. Place the grape seed oil, orange juice concentrate, salt, pepper, ginger, parsley and chives in a mini chopper or blender. Process until smooth and chill.

2. Preheat the oven to 425°F. Place a medium sized skillet in the oven.

3. Place the almonds in a small skillet over medium heat. Cook, tossing frequently, until slightly browned and remove from the heat.

4. Place the sesame seeds on a sheet of waxed paper. Place the chicken strips one at a time in the sesame seeds to coat just one side of each strip.

5. Remove the hot pan from the oven and spray lightly with olive oil. Place the chicken strips in the pan with the coated side down. Sprinkle the 1/8 teaspoon salt over the uncoated side and return the pan to the oven. After about 7 minutes turn the chicken strips over. The chicken will take another 8 - 10 minutes to cook.

6. While the chicken is cooking place the spinach in a large bowl with the chilled dressing. Toss until well coated. Divide between three plates. Sprinkle the mandarin oranges around the plate and then top with the toasted almonds and sliced red onion.

7. When the chicken is done place the strips on top of the salad and serve.

Baked Sweet Potatoes

http://allrecipes.com/recipe/baked-sweet-potatoes/detail.aspx

Yields: 4 servings

Ingredients

- 2 tablespoons olive oil

- 3 large sweet potatoes

- 2 pinches dried oregano

- 2 pinches salt & 2 pinches ground black pepper

Directions

1. Preheat oven to 350 degrees F (175 degrees C).

2. Coat the bottom of a glass or non-stick baking dish with olive oil, just enough to coat.

3. Wash and peel the sweet potatoes. Cut them into medium size pieces. Place the cut sweet potatoes in the baking dish and turn them so that they are coated with the olive oil.

4. Sprinkle moderately with oregano, and salt and pepper (to taste).

5. Bake in a preheated 350 degrees F (175 degrees C) oven for 60 minutes or until soft.

Boston Baked Beans

http://allrecipes.com/recipe/boston-baked-beans/detail.aspx

Yields: 6 servings

Ingredients

- 2 cups navy beans

- ½ pound bacon

- 1 onion, finely diced

- 3 tablespoons molasses

- 2 teaspoons salt

- ¼ teaspoon ground black pepper

- ¼ teaspoon dry mustard

- ½ cup ketchup

- 1 tablespoon Worcestershire sauce

- ¼ cup brown sugar

Directions

1. Soak beans overnight in cold water. Simmer the beans in the same water until tender, approximately 1 to 2 hours. Drain and reserve the liquid.

2. Preheat oven to 325 degrees F (165 degrees C).

3. Arrange the beans in a 2 quart bean pot or casserole dish by placing a portion of the beans in the bottom of dish, and layering them with bacon and onion.

4. In a saucepan, combine molasses, salt, pepper, dry mustard, ketchup, Worcestershire sauce and brown sugar.

5. Bring the mixture to a boil and pour over beans. Pour in just enough of the reserved bean water to cover the beans. Cover the dish with a lid or aluminum foil.

6. Bake for 3 to 4 hours in the preheated oven, until beans are tender. Remove the lid about halfway through cooking, and add more liquid if necessary to prevent the beans from getting too dry.

Grilled Asparagus

http://allrecipes.com/recipe/grilled-asparagus/detail.aspx

Yields: 4 servings

Ingredients

- 1 pound fresh asparagus spears, trimmed
- 1 tablespoon olive oil
- Salt and pepper to taste

Directions

1. Preheat grill for high heat.
2. Lightly coat the asparagus spears with olive oil. Season with salt and pepper to taste.
3. Grill over high heat for 2 to 3 minutes, or to desired tenderness.

Sesame Green Beans

http://allrecipes.com/recipe/sesame-green-beans/detail.aspx

Yields: 4 servings

Ingredients

- 1 tablespoon olive oil

- 1 tablespoon sesame seeds

- 1 pound fresh green beans, cut into 2-inch pieces

- ¼ cup chicken broth

- ¼ teaspoon salt

- Freshly ground black pepper to taste

Directions

1. Heat oil in a large skillet or wok over medium heat. Add sesame seeds. When seeds start to darken, stir in green beans.

2. Cook, stirring, until the beans turn bright green.

3. Pour in chicken broth, salt and pepper. Cover and cook until beans are tender-crisp, about 10 minutes.

4. Uncover and cook until liquid evaporates.

Simple Pan-Seared or Grilled Corn

http://www.rachaelray.com/food/collections/lactose
/index.php?cat=fakeout

Ingredients

- Fresh corn on the cob – as many ears as you'd like to make

- Olive oil

- Salt

Directions

1. Husk the corn. Brush it lightly with olive oil and season with salt.

2. Heat a sauté pan or grill on medium-high heat. When hot, place the corn in the pan. Using tongs, rotate the corn every few minutes so that it browns all over.

3. Baste the corn with a little olive oil, as needed. If the corn is browning or charring too fast, lower the heat slightly. Cook for 7-10 minutes, until the corn is tender.

4. Eat the corn as-is, or cool to room temperature and slice the kernels from the cob and eat with a fork.

Mayo-less Egg Salad

http://www.rachaelray.com/recipe.php?recipe_id=41
49

Ingredients

- 3 tablespoons olive oil

- 2 tablespoons lemon juice

- 2 tablespoons Dijon mustard

- 6 hardboiled eggs

- 4 scallions, thinly sliced

- 1/2 bunch parsley, minced

- 6 oil-cured olives, pitted and minced

- Salt and freshly ground black pepper

Directions

1. In a small bowl, whisk together a dressing with the olive oil, lemon juice and mustard; set aside

2. In a large bowl, mash the eggs with a potato masher or a fork. Add the dressing along with the scallions, parsley and olives and fold in until well mixed. Season with salt and pepper.

Deviled Eggs

http://dairyfreecooking.about.com/od/fingerfoods/r
/devileggs.htm

Makes 20 deviled eggs

Prep Time: 10 minutes

Total Time: 10 minutes

Ingredients

- 10 large hard-boiled eggs, peeled and sliced in half

- ¼ cup plain fat-free soy mayonnaise

- ¼ cup dairy-free sour cream, either store-bought or homemade

- 1 T. Dijon mustard

- 2 T. finely chopped fresh chives or shallots (optional)

- Salt and pepper, to taste

- Paprika, for garnishing

Directions

1. Remove the yolks from the hard boiled eggs and
    transfer to a small mixing bowl, along with the soy
    mayonnaise, dairy-free sour cream, Dijon mustard,
    chives (if using), salt and pepper.

2. Mash well with a potato-masher or fork until the
    mixture is creamy. Scoop the yolk mixture into the
    egg whites and sprinkle with the paprika just before
    serving.

Desserts

Chocolate Pudding

http://silk.com/recipes/chocolate-pudding

Ingredients

- 1/3 cup unsweetened cocoa
- 3/4 cup sugar
- 1/4 tsp salt
- 1/4 cup cornstarch
- 3 cups Silk soy, almond or coconut milk, any flavor except Light
- 3 Tbsp margarine (or butter)
- 1 1/2 tsp vanilla

Directions

1. Combine the cocoa, sugar, salt and cornstarch in a saucepan and mix well.

2.   Slowly add the Silk, whisking constantly to prevent lumps. Bring this mixture to a boil over medium heat while whisking constantly.

3.   Lower the heat to a simmer, cover and simmer gently for 8-10 minutes, until pudding begins to thicken.

4.   Remove from the heat and whisk in the margarine (or butter) and vanilla.

5.   Pour into 1 large bowl or 8 small serving bowls and refrigerate for at least an hour until thoroughly chilled.

Lactose-Free Flourless Chocolate Cake

http://www.food.com/recipe/lactose-free-flourless-chocolate-cake-259374

Yields: 8 Servings

Ingredients

- 4 ounces unsweetened baking chocolate
- 1/2 cup canola oil
- 1 cup sugar
- 3 large eggs
- 1/2 cup unsweetened cocoa powder, plus additional for sprinkling

Directions

1. Preheat oven to 375°F and oil an 8-inch round baking pan. Line bottom with a round of wax paper.

2. Chop chocolate into small pieces. In a double boiler or metal bowl set over a saucepan of barely simmering water melt chocolate with oil, stirring, until smooth.

3. Remove top of double boiler or bowl from heat and whisk sugar into chocolate mixture. Add eggs and whisk well.

4. Sift 1/2 cup cocoa powder over chocolate mixture and whisk until just combined.

5. Pour batter into pan and bake in middle of oven 25 minutes, or until top has formed a thin crust.

6. Cool cake in pan on a rack 5 minutes and invert onto a serving plate.

Lactose-Free Cheesecake

http://www.food.com/recipe/lactose-free-cheesecake-257731

Ingredients

Yields: 8 servings

- 6 ounces Keebler reduced-fat pie crusts
- 1 (12 ounce) package soft tofu
- 1/2 cup Lactaid calcium-fortified lactose-free skim milk
- 1/2 cup white sugar
- 1 tablespoon vanilla extract
- 1/4 cup maple syrup

Directions

1. Preheat oven to 350°F.
2. In a blender, combine tofu, milk, vanilla and syrup. Blend until smooth and pour into crust.
3. Bake for 30 minutes.
4. Remove from oven and cool. Refrigerate until chilled.

Vegan Chocolate Cola Brownies

http://dairyfreecooking.about.com/od/cookies/r/Vegan-Chocolate-Cola-Brownies.htm

If you don't have any dairy-free sour cream handy, simply replace it with applesauce or dairy-free soy yogurt.

Prep Time: 10 minutes

Cook Time: 35 minutes

Total Time: 45 minutes

Yield: 12-16 brownies

Ingredients

- 2 cups all-purpose flour

- 2 cups white granulated sugar

- 3/4 cup unsweetened cocoa powder

- 1 t. baking powder

- 1 t. salt

- 1 cup cola or other dark soda (not diet)

- 3/4 cup canola oil

- 1/4 cup dairy-free sour cream, such as Tofutti Sour Supreme

- 1 t. vanilla extract

- 1 cup dark dairy-free chocolate chips

Directions

1. Preheat the oven to 350.

2. Lightly oil a 9"x13" baking dish.

3. In a medium-large mixing bowl, combine the flour, sugar, cocoa powder, baking powder, and salt.

4. In another mixing bowl, whisk together the cola, canola oil, dairy-free sour cream and vanilla extract until well blended.

5. Add the wet ingredients to the dry, mixing until just combined.

6. Fold in the dairy-free chocolate chips.

1. Spread the batter evenly into the prepared dish and bake for 30-40 minutes or until the top cracks slightly.

2. Allow the brownies to cool completely in the pan before cutting into squares and serving.

Chocolate Cinnamon Bread Pudding

http://silk.com/recipes/chocolate-cinnamon-bread-pudding

Ingredients

- 2 large eggs
- 3 cups Silk Dark Chocolate almond milk
- 3 Tbsp brown sugar
- 2 Tbsp ground cinnamon
- 1 tsp pure vanilla extract
- Pinch of salt
- 8 oz lactose-free brioche or challah bread (about 8 1/2-inch slices), chopped into large pieces

Directions

1. Preheat oven to 375°F.

2. In a large bowl, beat eggs and then add almond milk, brown sugar, cinnamon, vanilla extract and salt, and whisk well.

3. Cut the bread into bite-sized pieces and place in an 8" x 8" nonstick casserole dish.

4. Pour the mixture slowly over the bread, ensuring you get it between all the pieces.

5. Cover with plastic wrap, refrigerate and soak for 30 minutes.

6. Bake 35-40 minutes, until set. Serve warm.

Strawberries with Balsamic Chocolate Sauce

http://www.drgourmet.com/recipes/desserts/strawber
rybalsamicchocolate.shtml

Servings = 2 | Serving size =1/2 pint strawberries with 1
Tbsp. balsamic chocolate sauce

Cooking Time = 45 Minutes

This recipe can be multiplied by 2.

This recipe can be divided by 2.

This recipe makes enough balsamic chocolate sauce for 8
servings.

Ingredients

- 1 cup balsamic vinegar

- 2 ounces bittersweet chocolate (crumbled)

- 1 pint fresh strawberries (rinsed, stemmed and
  sliced)

- 1 tsp sugar

Directions:

1. Place the balsamic vinegar in a small stainless steel or non-reactive sauce pan over medium heat. When the vinegar comes to a boil reduce the heat so that the liquid is simmering. Cook for about 30 - 40 minutes until reduced to 1/4 cup.

2. Cool slightly and then add the chocolate. Whisk until the chocolate is melted and let cool for about 30 minutes.

3. While the vinegar is reducing combine the sliced strawberries and sugar in a bowl and toss until well blended. Refrigerate for at least an hour.

4. Divide the strawberries between two bowls when ready to serve. Top each serving with 1 tablespoon of the balsamic chocolate sauce.

Chocolate Cheesecake with Hints of Orange (Lactose-Free)

http://www.rachaelray.com/food/collections/lactose/index.php?cat=desserts

Serves 6

Ingredients

For the crust:

- 3 cups graham crackers (Annie's brand Honey Bunny Grahams are dairy-free)
- 1/4 cup unrefined coconut oil, at room temperature

For the filling:

- 6 ounces dark chocolate (lactose-free)
- 1 cup sugar
- 3 tablespoons unrefined coconut oil, at room temperature
- 1 teaspoon vanilla extract
- Zest of 1 organic orange
- 3 tablespoons orange juice

- 1/4 teaspoon salt

- Optional: orange slices and cocoa nibs, for garnish

Directions

1. Pre-heat the oven to 350°F.

2. Place the graham crackers and coconut oil in the bowl of a food processor and grind until they form a coarse meal that clumps together easily.

3. Lightly oil a 10-inch round springform pan. Press the crust evenly over the bottom of the pan and up the sides to a height of 1 1/2 inches. Bake for 10 minutes, or until the crust turns golden. Let cool to room temperature.

4. Melt the chocolate over a double-boiler. Add the sugar and coconut oil and stir until smooth. Remove from the heat and cool to room temperature.

5. Puree the tofu in the bowl of a food processor. Add the chocolate, vanilla, orange zest and juice and salt. Puree until smooth.

6. Pour the filling into the prepared crust and smooth the top. Cover with parchment paper or plastic wrap and chill in the refrigerator for 4-6 hours, until firm.

7. Slice and serve with orange slices and cocoa nibs, if desired.

Mango-Banana Ice Cream (Lactose Free)

http://www.rachaelray.com/recipe.php?recipe_id=45 50

Makes 3 cups

Ingredients

- 1 cup frozen banana chunks
- 2 cups frozen mango chunks
- 3 tablespoons coconut milk
- 2 tablespoons honey
- A pinch of salt

Directions

Place all ingredients except the coconut flakes in a food processor and puree until smooth. Transfer to a sealed, airtight container and chill in the freezer for 30 minutes to firm up the ice cream. Serve garnished with coconut flakes.

Blueberry Pie

http://www.rachaelray.com/recipe.php?recipe_id=43
15

Serves 12

Ingredients

2 frozen 9-inch pie crusts (I prefer Oronoque Orchards
Homestyle Pie Crust)

4 cups frozen blueberries

1 teaspoon almond extract

2 tablespoons tapioca pearls

1/2 cup sugar

A pinch of salt

1/2 teaspoon cinnamon

1 teaspoon grated lemon zest

Cinnamon-sugar, for dusting

Directions

1. Pre-heat the oven to 400° F.

2. Place one of the pie crusts into a glass pie plate. If
   it cracks, don't fret, just pinch the dough together
   to cover up the cracks.

3. In a mixing bowl, combine the blueberries, almond extract, tapioca, sugar, salt, cinnamon and zest. Stir. Immediately spoon the filling into the crusted pie plate and even out with the back of your spoon.

4. Take the second crust and place over the pie so that it is covered. Pinch the ends of the pie together and poke holes all over the center of the pie. If you have rips and tears in the dough, that's good – you need the pie to have some breathing room.

5. Dust the pie with cinnamon-sugar and pop in the oven for 30 minutes, then turn the oven down to 350° F and let it cook for another 30 minutes. If the crust is starting to darken too much, your pie is most likely done.

6. Take the pie out and allow to cool for at least 3 hours on a cooling rack. It needs to set, so do not cut it before it's ready!

Carob Pudding

http://www.rachaelray.com/recipe.php?recipe_id=28
23

Serves 2 - 4

Ingredients

- 2 ripe avocadoes

- 6 tablespoons unsweetened carob powder

- 1/2 cup plus 2 tablespoons maple syrup

- 3 tablespoons freshly squeezed lemon juice

- 2 teaspoons vanilla extract

- 1/4 teaspoon salt

- 1/4 teaspoon ground nutmeg

- 1-2 ripe bananas (optional)

- 1/4 cup chopped nuts (optional)

Directions

1. Place all of the ingredients except the bananas and nuts in the bowl of a food processor and process until smooth. Chill for 1 hour before serving.

2. To serve, spoon some of the pudding into a bowl or glass. Thinly slice the banana and place several slices on top. Top with chopped nuts if desired.

Almond Paste Cookies

http://www.rachaelray.com/recipe.php?recipe_id=37
51

Makes approximately 8 dozen cookies

Ingredients

- 2 pounds almond paste

- 1 2/3 cups granulated sugar

- 3 cups confectioners' sugar

- 1 teaspoon salt

- 6 rounded tablespoons cornstarch

- 1 cup egg whites

- 1 ½ pounds blanched, slivered/sliced almonds

Directions

1. Grate the almond paste with the large holes of a box grater.

2. Mix the sugars and cornstarch together in a large bowl. Add the grated almond paste to the sugar mixture. Mix until fine granules form (you can also do this in a mixer on low).

3. Beat the egg whites in a separate bowl with a fork until frothy, 1-2 minutes. Add the egg whites and salt to the sugar/almond paste mixture and mix to combine.

4. Roll the dough into teaspoon-size balls and roll in the slivered/sliced almonds to coat. The dough will be very loose – keep your hands wet to make it easier to roll.

5. Place the balls on wax or parchment paper and cover with additional paper. Let the dough balls sit out on the countertop for 1-3 hours, until they dry out a bit.

6. Pre-heat the oven to 375°F.

7. Bake the cookies on parchment paper-lined cookie sheets for 12-15 minutes, until puffed and light golden brown.

Note: This recipe may be halved.

Very Berry Smash with Meringues and Sorbet

http://www.rachaelray.com/recipe.php?recipe_id=41 08

Serves 4

Ingredients

- 1/2 cup strawberries, sliced
- 1/2 pint blackberries
- A handful of blueberries
- A handful of raspberries
- A few fresh mint leaves, chopped
- A couple of fresh basil leaves, torn
- 2 shots limoncello liqueur *or* 3 tablespoons simple syrup
- 1 pint lemon sorbet
- 4 plain (vanilla) store-bought meringue nests

Directions

1. Mash the berries and herbs with the limoncello or syrup in a bowl with a potato masher or fork. Let stand for 5 minutes.

2. Scoop the sorbet into serving bowls and add the meringues. Pour the berry mash on top.

Apple Pot Pies

http://www.rachaelray.com/recipe.php?recipe_id=30
73

Serves 4

Ingredients

- 6 tart apples, such as Granny Smith *or* Northern Spies, peeled, seeded and diced

- 1/2 cup dried sweetened cranberries (a couple of handfuls)

- 1/2 cup dark brown sugar

- 1 teaspoon ground ginger

- 2 teaspoons ground cinnamon

- 1 teaspoon freshly grated nutmeg

- Juice of 1 lemon

- A pinch of salt

- 1 pie dough

- 1 egg, lightly beaten

- 4 ceramic or oven-safe individual glass bowls *or* large ramekins

Directions

1. Pre-heat the oven to 400°F.

2. In a mixing bowl, combine the apples, cranberries, brown sugar, ginger, cinnamon, nutmeg, lemon juice and salt.

3. Roll out the pie dough and cut out four rounds that are slightly larger than the mouth of the baking dishes.

4. Fill the dishes with the apple mixture. Top each ramekin with a round of pie dough and crimp the edges with the tines of a fork. Brush the crust with the egg wash.

5. Transfer the baking dishes to a baking sheet. Bake until the crust is golden brown and the apples are tender, about 20-30 minutes.

6. Serve warm or at room temperature plain or topped with vanilla ice cream or whipped cream.

Crunchy Monkey Peanut Butter-Banana Sticks

http://www.rachaelray.com/recipe.php?recipe_id=16 18

Ingredients

- 1/2 cup chunky-style peanut butter

- 2 tablespoons honey (a couple of drizzles)

- 1 cup fancy granola with nuts and raisins

- 2 large bananas

Directions

1. Heat the peanut butter in the microwave on high for 20 seconds to loosen it, then stir the honey into it.

2. Place the granola into a food processor and lightly process to crush up the granola, nuts and raisins.

3. Peel and cut each banana in half across the middle. Insert a popsicle or chopstick into the cut end of each half-banana. Spread one side of each banana stick with 1/4 of the peanut sauce, then coat liberally with spoonfuls of granola, gently pressing it into the peanut butter. Eat right off the sticks!

Chocolate Hazelnut Crepes

http://silk.com/recipes/chocolate-hazelnut-crepes

- 1 1/4 cup Silk Dark Chocolate almond milk

- 1 egg

- 1/3 cup chocolate hazelnut spread

- 1 cup flour

- 1/4 cup raw sugar or raw honey

- Fruit topping (like raspberries)

Directions

1. Whisk egg lightly. Add milk, chocolate hazelnut spread and sugar (or honey), whisking until combined thoroughly.

2. Blend in flour, scraping the sides of bowl until well combined. Let sit for about five minutes to thicken a little. Consistency should resemble heavy cream.

3. Heat an 8" skillet on medium-high and spray with cooking spray or grease lightly. Pour about 1/4-1/2 cup of batter into heated pan, sliding the pan around gently in a circle until batter spreads evenly.

4. Cook until the bottom is heated through and the edges begin to harden while bubbles form on top, about 45-60 seconds.

5. Using a spatula, slide gently to the side and flip.

6. Cook another 30-45 seconds, flip once more to ensure crepe is cooked thoroughly, and slide onto a plate.

7. Serve warm with fresh fruit.

Lactose-free Vanilla Panna Cotta with Balsamic Strawberries

http://www.lowfodmap.com/lactose-free-vanilla-panna-cotta-balsamic-strawberries/

Yield: Serves 6

Panna Cotta means "cooked cream" in Italian, and, for those of us with lactose intolerance, it would normally be the sort of dessert to avoid. However, with the great range of lactose-free dairy products available, that doesn't have to be the case. The key to this dessert is to use real vanilla, either a vanilla bean or vanilla bean paste which are both readily available in supermarkets; please don't settle for essence or even extract for this one.

The panna cotta should be made a day in advance so that it sets properly. You can use molds, ramekin dishes, or whatever you have in your kitchen—such as tea cups, drinking glasses, wine glasses or a muffin tins. Fifteen minutes before serving, mix the sliced strawberries with some icing sugar and balsamic vinegar and let it meld. Then top the pudding with the mixture.

Ingredients:

- 1 ½ cups reduced-fat, lactose-free cream (long-life milk aisle)

- 1 ½ cups (375ml) reduced-fat lactose-free milk

- 1 vanilla bean, split lengthways and seeds scraped out

- 1/3 (75g) cup castor sugar

- 2 ½ teaspoons gelatin

- 2 tablespoons cold water

- 150g strawberries, washed and hulled

- 2 teaspoons icing sugar mixture

- ¾ teaspoon balsamic vinegar

Directions:

Day 1:

1. Combine the cream, milk, vanilla bean and seeds in a saucepan and bring almost to the boil (keep a close eye on it)

2. Remove from the heat and stand for 15 minutes to allow the vanilla to infuse.

3. Add the sugar and warm gently over low heat to dissolve; remove from the heat.

4. Sprinkle the gelatin over the cold water in a small heatproof bowl or teacup.

5. Fill a small saucepan with water to a depth of approximately 3cm. Bring to the boil, remove from the heat, then sit the bowl of gelatin in the saucepan of hot water, stirring the gelatin until it's dissolved.

6. Stir the gelatin into the vanilla-infused cream.

7. Choose 6 molds that will hold at least ½ cup (125ml) and lightly grease with oil.

8. Strain the cream mixture into a jug then divide evenly between the molds. Chill the panna cotta in the fridge overnight.

Day 2:

1. Fifteen minutes before you are ready to serve, slice the strawberries and mix with the icing sugar and balsamic vinegar; set aside.

2. To unmold the panna cotta, run a knife around the edge of the mold, cover with a serving plate, then turn over and remove the mold (they might need a little tap and wriggle to release).

3. Divide the balsamic strawberries amongst each plate, arranging on top and beside each panna cotta.

4. *Tip: Wash and dry the vanilla pod after making the panna cotta. Cut into 4 pieces and place in a jar with a couple of cups sugar and seal. After a week or so you will have vanilla scented sugar to add to coffee, sprinkle over a tea cake or whatever else comes to your imagination.

Super Nutty Cookies (Wheat Free-Lactose Free)

http://www.food.com/recipe/super-nutty-cookies-wheat-free-lactose-free-106438

Yields: 24 Servings

Ingredients:

- 1 cup almond butter or 1 cup peanut better
- 1 cup packed brown sugar
- 1 large egg
- 1 teaspoon baking soda

Directions:

1. Preheat oven to 350 degrees

2. Combine all ingredients in a medium sized bowl, using a wooden spoon or heavy duty mixer.

3. After thoroughly mixed add any additional optional ingredients—cracked nuts, chocolate chips, or carob chips.

4. Roll into very small balls and place 2 inches apart on cookie sheet

5. Bake 9 minutes in the oven or until puffed and golden. Cookies will be soft until cooled off.

Frozen Fruit Cups

http://www.food.com/recipe/frozen-fruit-cups-278998

Yields: 16 one-cup servings

Ingredients

- 16 ounces frozen sweetened strawberries, thawed
- 12 ounces pineapple-orange juice concentrate, thawed
- 2 (20 ounce) cans crushed pineapple, undrained
- 2 (11 ounce) cans mandarin oranges, undrained
- 6 bananas, diced (yellow but not too ripe)
- 1/3 cup lemon juice (bottled is fine)
- 16 ounces frozen blueberries

Directions

1. Combine all ingredients in a very large bowl.
2. Freeze in 1-cup increments.
3. Thaw slightly before serving, to a slushy consistency.

Lactose-Free Milk Shake

http://www.food.com/recipe/lactose-free-milk-shakes-482071

Ingredients

Yields: 2 servings

- 2 cups lactose-free milk (like Lactaid whole milk)

- 8 ounces Cool Whip, free (half container)

- 2-4 tablespoons chocolate (to taste) or 2-4 tablespoons strawberry syrup (to taste)

Directions:

1. Blend the frozen Cool-whip FREE, lactose-free milk and syrup until the Cool-whip is incorporated.

2. Churn until it's thick enough to eat by spoon.

3. Then add toppings: fruit, candy, cookies, etc.

Strawberry Milkshake

http://www.rachaelray.com/recipe.php?recipe_id=45
65

Makes 3 Cups

Ingredients

- 3 tablespoons coconut flakes

- 1/4 cup raw cashews

- 4 pitted dates

- 1 1/2 cups cold water

- 1 1/2 cups frozen strawberries

- 1/4 teaspoon vanilla extract

- 1/4 teaspoon cinnamon

Directions

Place the coconut flakes, cashews, dates and water in a
blender and soak for 30 minutes. Add the strawberries,
vanilla and cinnamon and blend until smooth.

References & Resources

Books

Hobbs, Suzanne Havala *Living Dairy Free for Dummies* (Indiana: Wiley Publishing, Inc., 2010) **)** [Accessed 25 June 15, 2011]

Northrup, M.D., Christiane *The Wisdom of Menopause* (Batam, 2001)[Accessed 25 January 15, 2013]

Web

Lactose Intolerance

http://digestive.niddk.nih.gov/ddiseases/pubs/lactoseinto
lerance/#top [Accessed 14 June 2011]

http://www.mayoclinic.com/health/vitamin-
d/NS_patient-vitamind/DSECTION=dosing   [Accessed
15 October 2012]

Lactose Intolerance - Topic Overview

http://www.webmd.com/digestive-disorders/tc/lactose-
intolerance-topic-overview [Accessed 14 June 2011]

Lactose Intolerance - Topic Overview, Part 2

http://www.webmd.com/digestive-disorders/tc/lactose-
intolerance-topic-overview?page=2   [Accessed   14   June
2011]

Lactose Intolerance - Topic Overview, Part 3

http://www.ohsu.edu/xd/health/services/doernbecher/p
atients-families/topic-by-
id.cfm?ContentTypeId=85&ContentId=P00388&WT_ran
k=4 [Accessed 25 July 2012]

National Digestive Diseases Information Clearinghouse

www.digestive.niddk.nih.gov[AccessedFebruary 28, 2011.

Lactase

http://www.webmd.com/hw-popup/lactase
[Accessed 14 June 2011]

Lactose Intolerance - Exams and Tests

http://www.webmd.com/digestive-disorders/tc/lactose-intolerance-exams-and-tests [Accessed 14 June 2011]

Lactose Intolerance - Treatment Overview

http://www.webmd.com/digestive-disorders/tc/lactose-intolerance-treatment-overview [Accessed 14 June 2011]

Lactose Intolerance Treatment Overview, Part 2

http://www.webmd.com/digestive-disorders/tc/lactose-intolerance-treatment-overview?page=2 [Accessed 14 June 2011]

Lactose Intolerance -Treatment Overview, Part 3

http://www.webmd.com/digestive-disorders/tc/lactose-intolerance-treatment-overview?page=3 [Accessed 14 June 2011]

http://www.webmd.com/digestive-disorders/digestive-diseases-lactose-intolerance?page=2 [Accessed 5 November 2012]

Where is Lactose?

http://www.digestive.niddk.nih.gov/ddiseases/pubs/lactoseintolerance_ES/index.aspx#6 [Accessed 28 July 2012]

Supplements

http://ods.od.nih.gov/[Accessed 13 July 2012]

Calcium-Quick Facts

http://ods.od.nih.gov/factsheets/Calcium-QuickFacts/[Accessed 4 August 2012]

Calcium Requirements

http://ods.od.nih.gov/factsheets/Calcium-HealthProfessional/#h2 [accessed 4 August 2012]

http://www.livestrong.com/article/319464-a-lactose-restricted-diet/#ixzz2AvV6PCNz

http://www.cnn.com/2011/09/26/health/older-women-hip-fracture/index.html

Vitamin D Requirements

http://www.vitamindcouncil.org/about-vitamin-d/how-to-get-your-vitamin-d/uvb-exposure-sunlight-and-indoor-tanning/

http://www.sharp.com/nutrition/enough-vitamin-d.cfm

Non-milk Sources of Calcium

http://www.webmd.com/hw-popup/nonmilk-sources-of-calcium [Accessed 14 June 2011]

Tolerate Lactose Intolerance

http://www.webmd.com/food-recipes/features/tolerate-lactose-intolerance [Accessed 14 June 2011]

Could You Have Lactose Intolerance?

http://www.webmd.com/digestive-disorders/diagnosing [Accessed 14 June 2011]

Phosphorus

http://www.livestrong.com/article/474983-how-phosphorus-can-help-our-bodies/#ixzz25WkJjs1s

Not Just Dairy

http://www.webmd.com/digestive-disorders/diagnosing?page=2 [accessed 14 June 2011]

American Dietetic Association

www.eatright.org [accessed February 28, 2011.]

Challenges for a Dairy-Free Diet

http://www.bbc.co.uk/food/diets/dairy_free   [Accessed 14 June 2011]

Percentages of lactose

http://www.stevecarper.com/li/list_of_lactose_percentages.htm [Accessed 31 October 2012]

Where is Lactose?

www.lactaid.com

http://www.digestive.niddk.nih.gov/ddiseases/pubs/lactoseintolerance_ES/index.aspx#6 [accessed 28 July 2012]

Lactose limits

http://www.webmd.com/digestive-disorders/lactose-intolerance-12/slideshow-dairy October 2012 [accessed 31]

Lactose Intolerance Index

http://my.clevelandclinic.org/disorders/lactose_intolerence/hic_lactose_intolerance.aspx

Kefir

http://lifeway.net/LifewayWorld/KefirProbiotics/Kefir.aspx[accessed 5 November 2012]

Healthy Yogurt

http://www.lucyskitchenshop.com/yogourmet.html

http://www.youtube.com/watch?v=DQL4h8DLrmY

Fast Foods

Big Mac: Lactose

http://nutritiondata.self.com/foods-
000012000000000000000-
4w.html#ixzz2C7ve7fBN[accessed 13 November 2012]

Kentucky Fried chicken

http://www.livestrong.com/article/411541-lactose-
restricted-diets-and fast-foods/

Bugler King, Vanilla Shake Lactose: 4260mg

http://nutritiondata.self.com/foods-
000012000000000000000-1w.html?[accessed 13 November
2012]

McDonald's Quarter Pounder

http://nutritiondata.self.com/foods-
021012000000000000000-3w.html?[accessed 13 November
2012]

Lactose Levels of Popular Dairy Foods

 http://www.circleofmoms.com/article/lactose-levels-
popular-dairy-foods-01535#_

Yogurt and dairy allergies

http://www.livestrong.com/article/323738-yogurt-for-lactose-intolerant-people/#ixzz2CFAUbEhw

Eating out

http://www.godairyfree.org/eating-out

Kosher food and lactose intolerance

http://www.ehow.com/facts_4970271_definition-kosher-food.html#ixzz2CawBtrC0

http://http://www.ehow.com/how_12303_keep-kosher.html#ixzz2CayvCP8f

http://www.ehow.com/list_5984013_list-common-kosher-foods.html#ixzz2CbFdaCQP

http://en.wikipedia.org/wiki/Kosher_foods

http://www.ehow.com/list_7255719_kosher-restaurants-florida.html

http://www.amazon.com/Kosher-Clueless-but-Curious-Fact-Filled/dp/1881927318

http://www.jta.org/

Calcium

http://www.livestrong.com/article/319464-a-lactose-restricted-diet/#ixzz2AvV6PCNz

http://www.livestrong.com/article/482169-what-are-the-causes-of-human-calcium-depletion/#ixzz2DXNwQKZm

Resistance training

http://www.emedicinehealth.com/strength_training/article_em.htm

Celiac disease

http://www.wellsource.info/wn/ask-celiac.pdf

Crohn's disease

http://www.crohnsonline.com/what-is-crohns-disease/default.aspx?cid=ppc_ppd_hum_ggl_gastro_9614

Ulcerative colitis

http://www.nlm.nih.gov/medlineplus/ulcerativecolitis.html

Bone Density Test

http://www.livestrong.com/article/28869-bone-density-test-performed/#ixzz2Sie2DdDr

Lactose in medications

http://www.medicalfaq.net/can_you_become_lactose_intolerant_/ta-75533/p6

Food Diaries

http://skygazerlabs.com/wp/

Food Allergy Detective

http://www.foodallergydetective.com/

Supplements

Vitamin B6

http://ods.od.nih.gov/factsheets/VitaminB6HealthProfessional/B 12

Vitamin B 12

http://ods.od.nih.gov/factsheets/VitaminB12-HealthProfessional/

Folic acid

http://ods.od.nih.gov/factsheets/FolateHealthProfessional/"

Recipes

Easy Granola

http://www.drgourmet.com/recipes/breakfast/easygranola.shtml

Pumpkin Bread

http://www.rachaelray.com/recipe.php?recipe_id=4556

Holiday Brunch Gus-tinis

http://www.rachaelray.com/recipe.php?recipe_id=2388

Bacon Garlic Hash Browns

http://www.drgourmet.com/recipes/breakfast/baconhash
br

Healthy Fresh Orange Coconut Muffins

http://www.food.com/recipe/healthy-fresh-cranberry-
orange-coconut-muffins-489471

Dairy-Free Banana Muffins

http://dairyfreecooking.about.com/od/muffinsbiscuits/r/
DairyFree_Banana_Muffins_Recipe.htm

Zucchini Cranberry Muffins

http://www.rachaelray.com/recipe.php?recipe_id=4228

Pumpkin Oatmeal

http://low-cholesterol.food.com/recipe/pumpkin-
oatmeal-102176

French Toast (gluten-free, lactose & casein-free)

http://www.food.com/recipe/french-toast-gluten-free-
lactose-casein-free-203497

Gluten-and lactose-free bread

http://www.food.com/recipe/gluten-lactose-free-bread-
57170

Healthy Squash Bread

http://www.rachaelray.com/recipe.php?recipe_id=4148

Non-Dairy/Lactose-Free/Vegan "cheese"

http://www.food.com/recipe/non-dairy-lactose-free-vegan-cheese-164469

Butternut Squash Carrot Avocado Almond Salad (gluten- and lactose-free)

http://www.food.com/recipe/butternut-squash-carrot-avo-almond-salad-gluten-lactose-free-330873

Grilled Mediterranean Chicken (or Tofu) and Grape Skewers

http://www.godairyfree.org/recipes/grilled-mediterranean-skewer-recipe

Cheese Pizza with Basil Leaves

http://www.rachaelray.com/recipe.php?recipe_id=4557

Mexican Fiesta Dairy-Free or Vegan Pizza

http://www.godairyfree.org/recipes/entrees/dairy-free-mexican-vegan-pizza

Baked Sweet Potatoes

http://allrecipes.com/recipe/baked-sweet-potatoes/detail.aspx

BBQ Pork for Sandwiches—Slow Cooker Pulled Pork

http://allrecipes.com/recipe/bbq-pork-for-sandwiches/detail.aspx

Lactose-Free Cheesy French Fries

http://dairyfreecooking.about.com/od/potatoes/r/CheesyFries.htm

Creamy Polenta with Sautéed Leafy Greens

http://www.rachaelray.com/recipe.php?recipe_id=4564

Yummy Honey Chicken Kabobs

http://allrecipes.com/recipe/yummy-honey-chicken-kabobs/detail.aspx

Sesame Green Beans

http://allrecipes.com/recipe/sesame-green-beans/detail.aspx

Grilled Asparagus

http://allrecipes.com/recipe/grilled-asparagus/detail.aspx

Spicy Tomato Soup Recipe

http://dairyfreecooking.about.com/od/soupschilistews/r/
Spicy_Tomato_Soup_Recipe.htm

Ginger-Soy Carrot Soup

http://www.rachaelray.com/recipe.php?recipe_id=3705

Creamy Tomato Soup

http://silk.com/recipes/creamy-tomato-soup

Lemongrass and Ginger Egg Drop Soup with Rainbow Chard

http://www.rachaelray.com/recipe.php?recipe_id=3955

Vegetable Posole (Mexican soup)

http://www.rachaelray.com/recipe.php?recipe_id=4494

Easy Baked Salmon with Wilted Spinach and Strawberry Salsa

http://www.godairyfree.org/recipes/salmon-recipe-
strawberry-salsa

Sesame Pasta Chicken Salad

http://allrecipes.com/recipe/sesame-pasta-chicken-
salad/detail.aspx

Pork Chops Smothered with Peppers and Onions

http://www.rachaelray.com/recipe.php?recipe_id=4466

Pork Stew with Fennel and Apricots

http://www.rachaelray.com/recipe.php?recipe_id=4499

Grilled Salmon

http://allrecipes.com/recipe/grilled-salmon-i/detail.aspx

Lactose-Free Indian Curry

http://www.food.com/recipe/lactose-free-indian-curry-479439

Pot Roast

http://www.drgourmet.com/recipes/maincourse/beef/potroast.shtml

Slow-Cooker Chicken Tortilla Soup

http://allrecipes.com/recipe/slow-cooker-chicken-tortilla-soup/detail.aspx

Creamy Butternut Squash Soup

http://silk.com/recipes/creamy-butternut-squash-soup

Chopped Nicoise Salad

http://www.drgourmet.com/recipes/salad/choppednicoise.shtml

Grilled Halibut with Tangerines and Capers

http://www.drgourmet.com/recipes/maincourse/fish/halibuttangerine.shtml

Maple Sage Turkey Breast

http://www.drgourmet.com/recipes/maincourse/chicken/maplesageturkey.shtml

Barbecue Shrimp Salad

http://www.drgourmet.com/recipes/salad/bbqshrimpsalad.shtml

Curried Shrimp and Coconut Rice Salad

http://www.drgourmet.com/recipes/salad/curriedshrimp.shtml

Green Beans in Walnut Vinaigrette

http://www.drgourmet.com/recipes/salad/greenbeanswalnutvin.shtml

Mediterranean Corn Salad

http://www.drgourmet.com/recipes/extras/medcornsalad.shtml

Curried Lentil Salad with Lamb

http://www.drgourmet.com/recipes/salad/curriedlentilla
mb.shtml

Citrus Vinaigrette

http://www.drgourmet.com/recipes/salad/citrusvinaigrett
e.shtml

Crab, Avocado and Mango Salad

http://www.drgourmet.com/recipes/salad/crabavocadom
ango.shtml

Spinach Salad with Ginger Dressing and Sesame Chicken

http://www.drgourmet.com/recipes/salad/sesamechicken
.shtml

Baked Sweet Potatoes

http://allrecipes.com/recipe/baked-sweet-
potatoes/detail.aspx

Boston Baked Beans

http://allrecipes.com/recipe/boston-baked-
beans/detail.aspx

Grilled Asparagus

http://allrecipes.com/recipe/grilled-asparagus/detail.aspx

Sesame Green Beans

http://allrecipes.com/recipe/sesame-green-beans/detail.aspx

Simple Pan-Seared or Grilled Corn

http://www.rachaelray.com/food/collections/lactose/index.php?cat=fakeout

Mayo-less Egg Salad

http://www.rachaelray.com/recipe.php?recipe_id=4149

Deviled Eggs

http://dairyfreecooking.about.com/od/fingerfoods/r/devileggs.htm

Chocolate Pudding

http://silk.com/recipes/chocolate-pudding

Lactose-Free Flourless Chocolate Cake

http://www.food.com/recipe/lactose-free-flourless-chocolate-cake-259374

Lactose-Free Cheesecake

http://www.food.com/recipe/lactose-free-cheesecake-257731

Vegan Chocolate Cola Brownies

http://dairyfreecooking.about.com/od/cookies/r/Vegan-Chocolate-Cola-Brownies.htm

Chocolate Cinnamon Bread Pudding

http://silk.com/recipes/chocolate-cinnamon-bread-pudding

Strawberries with Balsamic Chocolate Sauce

http://www.drgourmet.com/recipes/desserts/strawberrybalsamicchocolate.shtml

Chocolate Cheesecake with Hints of Orange (Lactose-Free)

http://www.rachaelray.com/food/collections/lactose/index.php?cat=desserts

Mango-Banana Ice Cream (Lactose Free)

http://www.rachaelray.com/recipe.php?recipe_id=4550

Blueberry Pie

http://www.rachaelray.com/recipe.php?recipe_id=4315

Carob Pudding

http://www.rachaelray.com/recipe.php?recipe_id=2823

Almond Paste Cookies

http://www.rachaelray.com/recipe.php?recipe_id=3751

Super Nutty Cookies (Wheat Free-Lactose Free)

http://www.food.com/recipe/super-nutty-cookies-wheat-free-lactose-free-106438

Very Berry Smash with Meringues and Sorbet

http://www.rachaelray.com/recipe.php?recipe_id=4108

Apple Pot Pies

http://www.rachaelray.com/recipe.php?recipe_id=3073

Crunchy Monkey Peanut Butter-Banana Sticks

http://www.rachaelray.com/recipe.php?recipe_id=1618

Chocolate Hazelnut Crepes

http://silk.com/recipes/chocolate-hazelnut-crepes

Lactose-free Vanilla Panna Cotta with Balsamic Strawberries

http://www.lowfodmap.com/lactose-free-vanilla-panna-cotta-balsamic-strawberries/

Super Nutty Cookies (Wheat Free-Lactose Free)

http://www.food.com/recipe/super-nutty-cookies-wheat-free-lactose-free-106438

Frozen Fruit Cups

http://www.food.com/recipe/frozen-fruit-cups-278998

Strawberry Milkshake

http://www.rachaelray.com/recipe.php?recipe_id=4565

Lactose-Free Milk Shake

http://www.food.com/recipe/lactose-free-milk-shakes-482071

Index

A

abdominal, 13, 29, 61
abdominal bloating, 304
adrenal exhaustion, 308
adrenal fatigue, 308
adrenal glands, 308
African, 23, 24, 67
Aging, 312
AIDS, 312
alcohol, 313
Alcohol, 304
allergic, 19, 62, 64
allergies, 299, 301
allopathic, 300, 303
almond, 16, 37, 43, 56, 79, 95, 132, 146, 163, 231, 238, 245, 246, 249, 250, 256, 262, 277
alternative health professionals, 302
ancestors, 25, 97
antacid, 108
antibiotics, 315, 316, 317
Antibiotics, 316
Apps, 58
arthritis, 92, 105
Asian, 23, 44, 67, 76
Asian cooking, 44
Asians, 24
autoimmune
    reaction, 304
autoimmune diseases, 300, 301

B

bacteria, 306, 307, 308, 314, 315, 316
Bacteria, 304
beneficial, 42, 43, 102
Big Mac, 44, 271
bloated, 31
bloating, 26, 29, 58

D

E

J

K

L

S

T

More Books by Regency Publications

Leaky Gut Syndrome
The Invisible Thief
That Steals Your Health and Wellbeing and
What to do about it!

Charlotte Alexander

Write eBooks: Make Money
The No-Fear Guide to Writing Your Own
Money-Spinning eBook

April Manning

Find them now on Amazon.

More about…

Leaky Gut Syndrome

The Invisible Thief
That Steals Your Health and Wellbeing and
What to do about it!

by Charlotte Alexander

Many people with lactose intolerance also suffer from leaky gut syndrome. Often the two go hand in hand. **Leaky Gut Syndrome** delivers straight talk on the causes and effects of this syndrome and how to heal it.

Could leaky gut syndrome be a health issue for you? Learn more about this syndrome as you strive for ultimate health and wellness.

[Excerpt]

Introduction:
The Thief Within

What if I told you there is an invisible thief that can enter your life and steal your wellbeing? This thief is a chameleon—with many identities—but always insidious and greedy. He is Leaky Gut. His loot? Your good health.

I was robbed by this devious thief and suffered with leaky gut syndrome for more than 20 years. I had no idea what was happening to me as I endured the nagging, chronic symptoms that seemed to take over my life.

My symptoms were many including: abdominal pain, irritable bowel syndrome, extreme allergies (I was diagnosed with 49 different ones), **lactose intolerance**, food intolerances, migraines, Candida, and dermatitis so severe that I had to wear two pairs of gloves to do the dishes—rubber gloves to protect me from the dishwater, and white cotton gloves inside the rubber gloves to protect me from the latex.

My unrelated symptoms were indeed a puzzle for allopathic (conventional) doctors. One told me it was all in my head, others prescribed medications that simply didn't work. Each tried to treat different symptoms, but never the underlying cause. I was misdiagnosed for many years.

What about you?

Has the same thing happened to you, too? Have you been suffering for far too long—visiting too many specialists—and spending a great deal of time and money? Have you felt like throwing your hands up in disgust and saying there's no hope of ever feeling better?

Don't give up! You and I both know that the failure of many conventional doctors to recognize and diagnose this disorder doesn't make it any less real.

There's help for you

It took me a long time to find a medical doctor to help me. I found a physician who specializes in integrated medicine (a healing-oriented medical approach that takes into account the whole of a person—the body, mind and spirit).

This doctor was the first to tell me about leaky gut syndrome and its effects. With his diagnosis, suddenly all my diverse symptoms made sense. The long-term result of a leaky gut is the development of autoimmune diseases, which means the body is attacking its own tissues. I indeed was suffering from various autoimmune diseases.

Your leaky gut

If you have leaky gut syndrome, you know the major toll it takes on your health and wellbeing. You know the limitations it puts on your body. Your symptoms may not be the same as mine; there are more than eighty recognized autoimmune diseases, including some as common as allergies, or as painful and stubborn as fibromyalgia. But whatever your chronic health issues and symptoms are, you know they're affecting your quality of life.

What if you could experience health, vitality and energy again?

That's what this book is all about. It's your personal resource and reference manual to help you understand the complexity of leaky gut syndrome. It's also chockfull of advice (that you can start using immediately) to help you identify and overcome this complex health concern.

I bet at some point, you too have probably been told that there is nothing basically wrong with you. If you've been on the same journey as I have, and haven't been able to find a solution, this book is indeed for you. I don't want anyone else to ever go through what I've been through—the twenty plus years of searching for help to feel better.

I've not only detailed what leaky gut is and what causes it, but I've even devoted a chapter to how your personal healthcare provider goes about making a definitive, accurate diagnosis.

You can have the quality of life you deserve. You just need the straight facts. You're going to get them **here!**

Diagnosis: The first step in healing

Once you have a diagnosis in hand, then leaky gut becomes far less mysterious and menacing. An accurate diagnosis also means the beginning of an effective treatment plan. Because, once you know you're suffering from leaky gut, you can take the necessary steps to overcome it.

And yes, I've provided you with a *variety* of ways that you can start healing your body. From diet to dietary supplements to herbs and beyond, you can choose the solutions that work for your specific, individual health problems.

Visit your healthcare provider before you begin

I have one word of caution. Before you embark on any program, you need to consult a healthcare provider. Look for medical doctors specializing in integrated medicine, as I did, or naturopathic physicians or other alternative health professionals to help guide you.

Make your best effort to find the right resources and the best fit for you. Finding the specific guidance you need is key. Your determination will be worth it. It's time to quit suffering and find something I suspect you haven't experienced in a long time…Hope.

Chapter 1
What Is Leaky Gut Syndrome?

L eaky what? If you've never heard the term before, you might be thinking it's a ridiculous name for a medical condition. Leaky gut syndrome (LGS) is also known as the more conventional-sounding "increased intestinal permeability."

But regardless of the name used to describe the condition, the fact is the allopathic (conventional) medical community, for the most part, refuses to acknowledge this far-too-common condition.

You'll need to look to medical doctors who specialize in integrated medicine, naturopathic physicians, or other natural healthcare practitioners who are experienced in treating leaky gut for help.

Picturing leaky gut

I'm going to describe leaky gut syndrome in detail. But before I do, it might be helpful to have a visual to make it easier to understand.

Imagine the lining of your small intestine like a window screen that lets air in and keeps bugs out. When leaky gut comes along, it punches holes in the screen.

Ever sit out on a screened porch at night? If mosquitoes can find a way through the screen, those nasty things will bite you. It's the same for your body. When the lining of your intestine becomes irritated and inflamed, the mucous lining of your small intestine becomes too porous (leaky).

Bacteria, other toxins, microorganisms, food particles and pathogens get into your blood stream, wreaking havoc. The presence of these toxins triggers an autoimmune reaction in which the immune system attacks your own cells. And this can eventually cause a host of gastrointestinal problems, not the least of which are abdominal bloating, excess gas and cramps.

But there are other ways this situation can affect your body as well, including causing fatigue, food sensitivities, and joint pain. Many of these so-called symptoms show up as a variety of conditions we consider disorders and diseases in and of themselves. Linking them to leaky gut syndrome is not usually what people think of doing. Listed below are just a handful of these symptoms:

Symptoms of leaky gut

- Alcohol use

- Autoimmune diseases

- Candida

- Certain medications

- Chronic constipation

- Chronic stress

- Environmental toxins

- Excessive consumption of processed foods

- Food sensitivities

- Low-fiber diet

- Low stomach acid

- Nutritional deficiencies

- Severe burns

Many times we treat these symptoms as disorders. We treat them, but don't realize why they exist to begin with. The truth of the matter is that, as the toxins in your blood take hold, they eventually affect other parts of your body, many of which are still banding together trying hard to keep you healthy.

Leaky gut syndrome and your liver

Among the first of your organs affected is your liver. The more toxins that enter your system, the more your liver works at excreting them. Yes, this does keep the organ active—very active. If left untreated, the liver gets overloaded and can no longer detoxify these materials. As a result, they're returned to the blood to circulate.

One of the tasks your blood performs is maintenance of something the medical community calls "chemical homeostasis." Through this mechanism, your body attempts to maintain an internal stability. It deftly coordinates the responses of various actions of different organs throughout your system. If, for any reason, the balance is disturbed, the poisonous chemicals and some physical debris get delivered to into what's called the tissue matrix.

Giving its all: the lymph system

And that's where another organ jumps into action, trying to maintain a healthy balance. It's your lymph system, a vital part of your immune system.

Even though your lymphatic system tries to collect and then neutralize these toxins, it isn't always successful. The burden is then placed on the liver and the tissue matrix, which have the potential to turn toxic.

It takes some time, but eventually what initially was merely a "gut-barrier" issue has escalated into tissue toxicity. And this, in turn, can trigger a chain reaction of other problems. If your tissue environment is compromised, bacteria grow.

Not only that, but the lymph fluids in your body accumulate causing lymphatic swelling. You'll soon recognize this by the presence of inflammation in your body. This swelling is what causes the multitude of possible symptoms, some of which go unexplained.

The consequences of toxin buildup

Let's take this situation one step further. If too many toxins accumulate, the immune system exhausts itself working against them. This means that, in all likelihood, a portion of the toxins inevitably enter the body. At the same time, the process also depletes your immune system.

You may wonder why the immune system is affected. It's a little known fact (and now one you're in on) that seventy percent of your immune system is actually located in and around your digestive system.

This portion of the system is called "gut-associated lymphatic tissues," or "GALT." These tissues are located in the lining of the digestive tract and in the intestinal mucus.

What happens when the liver is overwhelmed?

This condition can literally overwhelm your liver, leaving it unable to process everything efficiently. When this happens, the liver then turns to your immune system for help. Unfortunately, we've already established that your immune response is stressed, and unable to act as it should.

The bacteria then accumulate to unhealthy levels, and this opens the door for opportunistic infections to appear. These are infections you normally wouldn't develop. Due to the severely weakened state of your immune system, they "sneak in."

Another organ then becomes affected by this overrun of bacteria. Your adrenal glands, two small glands sitting atop each of your kidneys, are vital in resisting infection. The prolonged presence of leaky gut syndrome eventually — and slowly — reduces the healthy function of these glands as well.

In the initial stages, there is no adrenal excess. This can be easily tested by measuring your cortisol output—the hormone the adrenal glands produce. But, as the syndrome continues unabated, cortisol levels increase. And that's when a condition called "adrenal exhaustion" occurs.

Briefly, just a few of the symptoms indicating you may be experiencing adrenal fatigue include: exhaustion, sleep that doesn't refresh you, inability to cope with stress, difficulty concentrating and poor digestion.

How leaky gut syndrome reveals itself

Now that you understand — at least in general terms — how this syndrome develops, hopefully you have a greater appreciation for how all the parts of your body work together to help fight off disease. In the same way, your system teams up to create health. It's a two-way street.

It may not come as a surprise to you to discover that leaky gut syndrome can manifest itself in any number of ways in your system. While you can't call these "symptoms," they are indeed real health conditions. But the underlying cause of these conditions may very well be the presence of leaky gut syndrome.

In the next chapter, I discuss some of the factors that can cause leaky gut syndrome. Knowing what triggers this syndrome can help you take action to remedy it.

Chapter 2
The Causes of Leaky Gut Syndrome No One Talks About

By this time, you may have already approached a natural health practitioner or a naturopathic doctor who suspects that you may indeed have leaky gut syndrome. Probably your immediate question was, "What caused it?"

If only there were a simple one- or two-word answer to that question, but there isn't. In fact, there are a host of possible causes of this syndrome. And there are "hidden" causes that many don't even seem to talk about.

Therefore, if you're waiting for your healthcare provider to hand over one cause on a silver platter — well, unfortunately, that's not going to happen. More often than not, discovering the cause is sometimes the most difficult part of treating the syndrome.

Of course, you know your body better than anyone else. You know your health habits. And armed with this intimate information, when you're presented with a list of possible hidden causes, you may be able to identify the most likely causes for your body and check them out.

Common Causes of leaky gut syndrome

Here are just a few of the more common causes of this syndrome:

- Chronic use of NSAIDs

- Dysbiosis

- Candida

- Cancer therapy

- Chronic stress

- Environmental toxins

- Diet

- Aging

- Endotoxins

- AIDS

- Gastrointestinal disease

- Immune system overload

- Lack of Secretory IgA

- Abuse of alcohol

  • Trauma

  • Chronic infections

NSAIDs as a cause

NSAIDs (nonsteroidal anti-inflammatory drugs, (pronounced en-saids), are   medications used primarily to treat inflammation, mild to moderate pain, and fever.

They include such drugs as aspirin, Celebrex, ibuprofen, naproxen, Toradol, Lodine, Indocin, and more.

The success of NSAIDs lies in their ability to block tiny messengers known as *prostaglandins*. These substances circulate throughout your body and block pain and inflammation. But the work of these drugs doesn't end there.

The prostaglandins have another job. They're charged with healing and repairing your body. When you take an NSAID, you indeed are blocking the pain and giving yourself much-needed relief. But you're also effectively blocking any healing or repair process that needs to be performed.

That's right. Regardless of their tasks, though, the over-the-counter medication indiscriminately blocks all of the transmitters.

The digestive tract repairs itself every three days

The digestive tract repairs and replaces itself every three to five days. So you can see how the extended use of

NSAIDs blocks the needed repair process. Eventually, the lining of the tract weakens, becomes inflamed, and then leaks. And the result — you have leaky gut syndrome.

Not only that, but prolonged use of NSAIDs raises your risk of developing ulcers of the stomach and the duodenum.

Want more reasons to reduce your dependency on them? This class of medication causes bleeding, damage to the mucus membranes of your intestines and gastrointestinal inflammation.

Additionally, NSAID use can lead to colitis and relapses of ulcerative colitis. Who knew that these easily accessible, almost ubiquitous pills everyone takes with barely a second thought could be so potentially troublesome?

Dysbiosis

If you're like me, you've probably never heard of the term "dysbiosis." The word was created by Dr. Eli Metchnikoff, a 1908 Nobel Prize winner, for his work on friendly bacterial flora.

You're already aware of the need to keep a balance between the harmful or pathogenic bacteria — as they're called in the medical community — and the helpful bacteria, often called *flora.*

When this balance is disrupted and your body contains more harmful than friendly bacteria, this state is called dysbiosis. It's derived from the word *symbiosis,* which means "living in harmony" and the prefix *dys* which means "not."

Dr. Metchnikoff discovered the natural bacteria of yogurt can prevent and actually reverse bacterial infections. Not only that, but thanks to his research, he revealed that the bacteria in yogurt has the ability to displace quite a few organisms which produce disease. Additionally, the yogurt bacteria content could also reduce the amount of accompanying toxins.

Given the state of modern medicine at the turn of the 20th century, this represented an amazing advance in the treatment of bacterial infections.

With the advent of antibiotics and immunizations, though, his research seemed far less important and…well, quite frankly, outdated. Until recently, that is.

A host of new laboratory testing and corresponding research created a revival in the interest of the topic.

Menacing microbes and your health

Medical science is discovering microbes that don't belong in the digestive tract. And why is this of interest? The microbes very often form chemicals toxic to the cells which are located around them. But that's only part of the increase in interest. These microbes can also be a source of poison to you.

The overrun of microbes places the lining of your intestines at risk. The probable consequence? The creation of a vast array of potentially dangerous substances, including secondary bile acids, amines, phenols ammonia, indoles, and hydrogen sulfide.

In turn, these substances may damage your intestinal lining by injuring the brush borders. The brush borders are the largest manufacturer of digestive enzymes in your small intestine. Eventually the damaged brush borders enzymes may be absorbed into your bloodstream.

Unfortunately, the adverse toll they're taking on your body isn't recognized immediately. After a while they can cause chronic conditions, many of which never get diagnosed.

So what's the ultimate cause of dysbiosis? We've already talked about it: the overuse of medications. But the extended use of NSAIDs is only one trigger to the development of the buildup of bad bacteria. We'll discuss the other class of drugs which can trigger this state next.

Those antibiotics that get me well?

Surely you must be mistaken. Antibiotics help to improve my health. They cure my infections — all sorts of infections. I take them when I have swollen glands.

Well, you get the idea. They're a modern-day marvel.

Yes, I agree and there's where the problem comes in. The medical community has been depending on this type of medication for just about every ailment you can imagine. Most patients practically demand some sort of antibiotics when they walk into a doctor's office complaining of an ailment, even if they don't suffer from a bacterial infection. Doctors, for their part, readily agree.

When good antibiotics go bad...

[End of Preview]